THE COMPLETE DIABETIC COOKBOOK FOR BEGINNERS

The Easy Guide To 2000 Nutritious Days Of Super Easy & Healthy Diabetic Diet With A Complete Meal Plan Suitable For Prediabetic, Newly Diagnosed, Type 1 And 2 Diabetes

Nathan Wendy

Table of Contents

CHAPTER ONE 4

Understanding Diabetes and Nutrition 4

What is Diabetes and How Diet Affects It? 4

Types of Diabetes: Understanding the Differences..................7

Gestational Diabetes 8

Other Types of Diabetes 9

Basic Nutritional Guidelines for Diabetics 10

CHAPTER TWO 14

Setting the Foundation: Stocking Your Kitchen.................14

Essential Pantry Staples for Diabetic Cooking..................14

Must-Have Kitchen Equipment for Easy Meal Preparation 17

Understanding Sugar Substitutes and Healthy Alternatives....19

CHAPTER THREE 24

Breakfasts to Fuel Your Day 24

Quick and Healthy Breakfast Options for Busy Mornings 24

High-Fiber Breakfasts to Keep Blood Sugar Stable 27

Diabetic-Friendly Smoothies and Breakfast Casseroles...........29

Diabetic-Friendly Breakfast Casseroles.................................31

CHAPTER FOUR 33

Wholesome and Satisfying Lunches 33

Simple Salad and Wrap Recipes for Balanced Lunches 33

Protein-Packed Lunches to Keep You Full and Energized 36

Creative Lunch Ideas for Work or School 39

CHAPTER FIVE 42

Nourishing Dinners for Every Taste 42

Easy One-Pot Dinners for Weeknight Convenience 42

Flavorful Vegetarian and Plant-Based Dinner Options...........45

Comforting Slow Cooker and Instant Pot Recipes..................48

CHAPTER SIX 52

Smart Snacking Strategies...52

Nutrient-Dense Snack Ideas for Between Meals....................52

Homemade Snacks That Are Low in Sugar and High in Flavor.54

Portable Snacks for On-the-Go Convenience 57

CHAPTER SEVEN 60

Decadent Desserts Made Diabetic-Friendly...........................60

Lower-Sugar Dessert Recipes for Satisfying Sweet Cravings ...60

Indulgent Treats Made Healthier with Smart Ingredient Swaps
....65

CHAPTER EIGHT..68

Flavorful Side Dishes to Complement Any Meal 68

Simple Vegetable Side Dishes Packed with Nutrients 68

Whole Grain and Legume-Based Side Dishes for Balanced Nutrition........71

Creative Ways to Add Flavor to Your Side Dish Repertoire 74

CHAPTER NINE 77

Dining Out and Socializing with Diabetes 77

Strategies for Making Healthy Choices When Eating Out........77

Tips for Navigating Social Events and Celebrations.................80

Communicating Your Dietary Needs Effectively 82

CHAPTER TEN 84

Meal Planning and Preparation for Success............................84

Practical Tips for Meal Planning and Grocery Shopping.........84

Batch Cooking and Freezing Meals for Convenience..............87

Strategies for Portion Control and Balanced Eating 90

CHAPTER 11 94

DDIET FOR DIABETES 94

CHAPTER 12 132

31 DAYS MEAL PLAN 132

THE END..142

COPYRIGHT © 2023

CHAPTER ONE

Understanding Diabetes and Nutrition

What is Diabetes and How Diet Affects It?

Diabetes is a chronic condition characterized by high levels of glucose (sugar) in the blood. Glucose is the body's primary source of energy, and it comes from the food we eat. When we consume carbohydrates, they are broken down into glucose, which then enters the bloodstream. However, for glucose to be utilized by the body's cells, it requires insulin, a hormone produced by the pancreas.

In individuals with diabetes, there is either a lack of insulin production (Type 1 diabetes) or the body's cells become resistant to insulin (Type 2 diabetes). This results in elevated blood glucose levels, leading to various health complications if not managed properly. Diet plays a crucial role in managing diabetes because the types and amounts of foods consumed directly impact blood sugar levels.

Carbohydrates have the most significant effect on blood sugar levels because they are broken down into glucose during digestion. Therefore, people with diabetes need to monitor their carbohydrate intake carefully. Foods high in refined carbohydrates, such as white bread, pasta, sugary snacks, and sodas, can cause blood sugar spikes. On the other hand, complex carbohydrates found in whole grains, fruits, vegetables, and legumes are digested more slowly, resulting in a steadier rise in blood sugar levels.

Proteins and fats also affect blood sugar levels, albeit to a lesser extent than carbohydrates. Proteins are broken down into amino acids, some of which can be converted into glucose through a process called gluconeogenesis. Fats, especially unhealthy saturated and trans fats, can contribute to insulin resistance, worsening blood sugar control.

However, not all fats are detrimental to diabetes management. Healthy fats, such as those found in avocados, nuts, seeds, and oily fish, can improve insulin sensitivity and help stabilize blood sugar levels.

In addition to macronutrients, the timing and distribution of meals can also influence blood sugar control. Eating consistent meals and snacks throughout the day helps prevent dramatic fluctuations in blood sugar levels. Moreover, pairing carbohydrates with protein or healthy fats can slow down their absorption, preventing rapid spikes in blood sugar.

In summary, diet plays a crucial role in managing diabetes by directly impacting blood sugar levels. Monitoring carbohydrate intake, choosing complex carbohydrates over refined ones, and incorporating protein and healthy fats into meals can help stabilize blood sugar levels and improve overall health outcomes for individuals with diabetes.

Types of Diabetes: Understanding the Differences

Diabetes is a complex metabolic disorder characterized by elevated blood sugar levels. There are several types of diabetes, each with its unique causes, risk factors, and management strategies.

Type 1 Diabetes

Type 1 diabetes, formerly known as juvenile diabetes or insulin-dependent diabetes, is an autoimmune condition in which the immune system mistakenly attacks and destroys insulin-producing beta cells in the pancreas. As a result, the pancreas produces little to no insulin, leading to high blood sugar levels.

The exact cause of Type 1 diabetes is unknown, but it is believed to involve a combination of genetic predisposition and environmental triggers, such as viral infections or exposure to certain toxins.

Type 1 diabetes typically develops in childhood or adolescence, although it can occur at any age. It requires lifelong insulin therapy to regulate blood sugar levels. People with Type 1 diabetes must carefully monitor their blood sugar levels, adjust their insulin doses accordingly, and follow a balanced diet and exercise regimen to manage their condition effectively.

Type 2 Diabetes

Type 2 diabetes is the most common form of diabetes, accounting for approximately 90% of cases worldwide. It develops when the body becomes resistant to insulin or fails to produce enough insulin to meet its needs.

Unlike Type 1 diabetes, which is primarily an autoimmune condition, Type 2 diabetes is strongly associated with lifestyle factors such as obesity, physical inactivity, and unhealthy eating habits. Genetics also play a significant role in the development of Type 2 diabetes, with certain genetic variations increasing the risk of insulin resistance and impaired glucose metabolism.

Type 2 diabetes often develops gradually over time, with symptoms becoming apparent in adulthood. However, it is becoming increasingly prevalent in children and adolescents due to rising rates of obesity and sedentary lifestyles.

Initially, Type 2 diabetes can often be managed through lifestyle modifications, including dietary changes, regular exercise, and weight loss. However, as the condition progresses, oral medications and/or insulin therapy may be necessary to achieve and maintain adequate blood sugar control.

Gestational Diabetes

Gestational diabetes occurs during pregnancy and is characterized by high blood sugar levels that develop or are first recognized during pregnancy. It is caused by hormonal changes and increased insulin resistance, which occur naturally during pregnancy to ensure an adequate supply of glucose to the developing fetus.

Women who are overweight or obese, older than 25 years, have a family history of diabetes, or belong to certain ethnic groups (such as African American, Hispanic, Native American, or Asian) are at higher risk of developing gestational diabetes.

Gestational diabetes typically resolves after childbirth, but women who have had gestational diabetes are at increased risk of developing Type 2 diabetes later in life. Therefore, it is essential for women with a history of gestational diabetes to undergo regular screening for Type 2 diabetes and adopt healthy lifestyle habits to reduce their risk.

Other Types of Diabetes

In addition to Type 1, Type 2, and gestational diabetes, there are several other less common types of diabetes, including:

- **Monogenic Diabetes**: Caused by mutations in a single gene inherited from one or both parents. Monogenic diabetes includes maturity-onset diabetes of the young (MODY) and neonatal diabetes.

- **Secondary Diabetes**: Caused by underlying medical conditions or medications that impair insulin production or action. Examples include pancreatitis, cystic fibrosis-related diabetes, and steroid-induced diabetes.

Each type of diabetes requires personalized management strategies based on its underlying cause, severity, and individual factors such as age, overall health, and lifestyle habits. Effective management of diabetes involves a comprehensive approach that includes blood sugar monitoring, medication management, dietary modifications, regular exercise, stress management, and ongoing support from healthcare providers.

Basic Nutritional Guidelines for Diabetics

A healthy diet is essential for managing diabetes and preventing complications. Nutritional guidelines for diabetics focus on controlling blood sugar levels, promoting weight management, and reducing the risk of cardiovascular disease. Here are some basic nutritional guidelines for diabetics:

1. Carbohydrate Management

Carbohydrates have the most significant impact on blood sugar levels, so it's crucial for diabetics to monitor their carbohydrate intake. Carbohydrate counting is a common method used to manage blood sugar levels, where individuals track the number of grams of carbohydrates consumed in each meal and adjust their insulin doses accordingly.

Focus on consuming complex carbohydrates, such as whole grains, fruits, vegetables, and legumes, which are digested more slowly and cause a gradual rise in blood sugar levels. Limit the intake of refined carbohydrates, sugary snacks, and beverages, which can cause rapid spikes in blood sugar.

2. Portion Control

Controlling portion sizes is essential for managing blood sugar levels and promoting weight management. Use measuring cups, spoons, or visual cues to portion out appropriate serving sizes of carbohydrate-containing foods, protein sources, and fats.

Fill half of your plate with non-starchy vegetables, such as leafy greens, broccoli, cauliflower, and peppers, to increase fiber intake and promote satiety without significantly impacting blood sugar levels.

3. Balanced Meals and Snacks

Include a balance of carbohydrates, protein, and healthy fats in each meal and snack to help stabilize blood sugar levels and promote overall health. Pair carbohydrates with protein or healthy fats to slow down their absorption and prevent rapid spikes in blood sugar.

Choose lean protein sources, such as poultry, fish, tofu, legumes, and low-fat dairy products, to help control hunger and maintain muscle mass. Incorporate healthy fats, such as avocados, nuts, seeds, olive oil, and fatty fish, in moderation to support heart health and improve insulin sensitivity.

4. Fiber-Rich Foods

Include plenty of fiber-rich foods in your diet, such as whole grains, fruits, vegetables, legumes, nuts, and seeds. Fiber helps slow down the absorption of carbohydrates, regulate blood sugar levels, and promote digestive health.

Aim for at least 25 grams of fiber per day for women and 38 grams per day for men, but gradually increase fiber intake to avoid digestive discomfort. Drink plenty of water to help fiber move through the digestive tract smoothly and prevent constipation.

5. Limit Added Sugars and Processed Foods

Minimize the consumption of foods and beverages high in added sugars, such as sweets, desserts, sugary drinks, and processed snacks. These foods can cause rapid spikes in blood sugar levels and contribute to weight gain and poor overall health.

Read food labels carefully and choose products with minimal added sugars and simple ingredients. Opt for whole, unprocessed foods whenever possible and use natural sweeteners such as stevia, monk fruit, or erythritol in moderation if needed.

6. Stay Hydrated

Drink plenty of water throughout the day to stay hydrated and support optimal blood sugar control. Aim for at least eight 8-ounce glasses of water per day, or more if you're physically active or in a hot climate.

Limit the consumption of sugary beverages, caffeinated drinks, and alcohol, which can contribute to dehydration, weight gain, and fluctuations in blood sugar levels. Choose water, herbal tea, or unsweetened beverages as your primary sources of hydration.

7. Monitor Blood Sugar Levels

Regularly monitor your blood sugar levels using a blood glucose meter or continuous glucose monitor (CGM) to track how different foods and lifestyle factors affect your blood sugar levels. Keep a record of your blood sugar readings, meals, medication doses, physical activity, and other relevant factors to identify patterns and make informed adjustments to your diabetes management plan.

Consult with a registered dietitian or certified diabetes educator to develop a personalized meal plan tailored to your individual nutritional needs, lifestyle preferences, and health goals. Work collaboratively with your healthcare team to monitor your progress, adjust your treatment plan as needed, and address any concerns or challenges you may encounter along the way.

By following these basic nutritional guidelines for diabetics and adopting a healthy lifestyle, you can effectively manage your diabetes, improve your overall health and well-being, and reduce your risk of complications associated with the condition. Remember that consistency, balance, and moderation are key to long-term success in diabetes management.

CHAPTER TWO

Setting the Foundation: Stocking Your Kitchen

Essential Pantry Staples for Diabetic Cooking

Stocking your pantry with the right ingredients is essential for preparing nutritious and delicious meals that support blood sugar control. Here are some essential pantry staples for diabetic cooking:

1. **Whole Grains**: Opt for whole grain options such as brown rice, quinoa, oats, barley, and whole wheat pasta. These provide complex carbohydrates, fiber, and essential nutrients without causing rapid spikes in blood sugar levels.

2. **Legumes**: Include a variety of beans, lentils, and chickpeas in your pantry. Legumes are rich in protein, fiber, and complex carbohydrates, making them an excellent alternative to meat and a valuable addition to soups, salads, and main dishes.

3. **Canned Tomatoes and Tomato Products**: Stock up on canned diced tomatoes, tomato sauce, and tomato paste to add flavor and richness to sauces, stews, and casseroles. Look for low-sodium options to control your sodium intake.

4. **Healthy Oils**: Choose heart-healthy oils such as olive oil, avocado oil, and coconut oil for cooking, salad dressings, and

marinades. These oils provide essential fatty acids and can help improve insulin sensitivity.

5. **Herbs and Spices**: Keep a variety of herbs and spices on hand to add flavor to your meals without the need for excess salt, sugar, or fat. Options like garlic, ginger, cinnamon, cumin, paprika, and turmeric can enhance the taste of dishes while providing potential health benefits.

6. **Nuts and Seeds**: Incorporate unsalted nuts and seeds such as almonds, walnuts, chia seeds, and flaxseeds into your pantry for added texture, flavor, and nutritional value. These ingredients are rich in healthy fats, protein, fiber, and essential vitamins and minerals.

7. **Low-Sodium Broth or Stock**: Use low-sodium vegetable, chicken, or beef broth as a base for soups, stews, and sauces. Broth adds depth of flavor to dishes without contributing excessive sodium, making it a healthier option for diabetic cooking.

8. **Non-Starchy Vegetables**: Keep a variety of fresh, frozen, and canned non-starchy vegetables on hand, such as spinach, kale, broccoli, cauliflower, bell peppers, carrots, and zucchini. These vegetables are low in calories and carbohydrates but rich in fiber, vitamins, and minerals.

9. **Canned Fish and Seafood**: Stock up on canned tuna, salmon, sardines, and other seafood options packed in water or olive oil. Canned fish is convenient, affordable, and a good source of protein, omega-3 fatty acids, and essential nutrients.

10. **Low-Sodium Condiments and Sauces**: Choose low-sodium soy sauce, vinegar, mustard, hot sauce, and salsa to season and flavor your meals without excess salt or added sugars. These condiments add variety and complexity to dishes while keeping sodium intake in check.

By keeping these essential pantry staples on hand, you'll have the foundation for creating flavorful, nutritious meals that support your diabetes management goals. Be sure to check expiration dates regularly, rotate stock to use older items first, and plan meals based on what you have available in your pantry to minimize food waste.

Must-Have Kitchen Equipment for Easy Meal Preparation

Having the right kitchen equipment can make meal preparation more efficient, enjoyable, and stress-free. Here are some must-have kitchen tools and appliances for diabetic cooking:

1. **Quality Chef's Knife**: Invest in a sharp, high-quality chef's knife for slicing, dicing, and chopping fruits, vegetables,

meats, and herbs with precision and ease. A good knife makes meal prep faster and safer.

2. **Cutting Boards**: Use durable, non-porous cutting boards made of wood, plastic, or bamboo to protect your countertops and prevent cross-contamination when preparing raw ingredients. Consider having separate cutting boards for meat, poultry, seafood, and produce.

3. **Vegetable Peeler**: Keep a vegetable peeler on hand for peeling and trimming fruits and vegetables quickly and efficiently. Choose a comfortable, ergonomic design with a sharp blade for smooth peeling.

4. **Measuring Cups and Spoons**: Accurate measuring is crucial for portion control and achieving consistent results in cooking and baking. Invest in a set of measuring cups and spoons made of durable materials for precise ingredient measurements.

5. **Mixing Bowls**: Have a variety of mixing bowls in different sizes for mixing, whisking, marinating, and storing ingredients. Stainless steel, glass, or ceramic bowls are durable and easy to clean.

6. **Non-Stick Cookware**: Use non-stick pots and pans for cooking with minimal oil and easy cleanup. Choose high-

quality non-stick cookware that is free of harmful chemicals and durable enough to withstand regular use.

7. **Baking Sheets and Pans**: Have a selection of baking sheets, cake pans, muffin tins, and loaf pans for baking a variety of diabetic-friendly desserts, bread, and snacks. Opt for non-stick or silicone-coated bakeware for easy release and cleanup.

8. **Blender or Food Processor**: Invest in a blender or food processor for making smoothies, sauces, dips, purees, and soups. These versatile appliances can also be used to chop, shred, and blend ingredients for quick and convenient meal preparation.

9. **Slow Cooker or Instant Pot**: Consider adding a slow cooker or Instant Pot to your kitchen arsenal for hands-off cooking and meal prep. These appliances are ideal for making soups, stews, chili, braised meats, and one-pot meals with minimal effort.

10. **Digital Kitchen Scale**: Use a digital kitchen scale for accurate portion control and ingredient measurements, especially when following recipes or tracking macronutrients. A scale helps ensure consistency and precision in cooking and baking.

By equipping your kitchen with these essential tools and appliances, you'll be well-prepared to tackle diabetic cooking with confidence and ease. Invest in high-quality, durable equipment that suits your cooking style and preferences, and prioritize items that will help streamline meal preparation and support your health goals.

Understanding Sugar Substitutes and Healthy Alternatives

Sugar substitutes, also known as artificial sweeteners or sugar alternatives, are substances used to sweeten foods and beverages without adding calories or significantly impacting blood sugar levels. Understanding the different types of sugar substitutes and their potential health effects can help individuals with diabetes make informed choices about sweeteners and incorporate them into their diet in moderation.

1. Artificial Sweeteners

Artificial sweeteners are synthetic sugar substitutes that provide sweetness without calories. They are much sweeter than table sugar (sucrose) and are used in smaller quantities to achieve the desired level of sweetness. Some common artificial sweeteners include:

- **Aspartame**: Sold under brand names such as NutraSweet and Equal, aspartame is commonly used in diet sodas, sugar-free desserts, and tabletop sweeteners. It is heat-stable and suitable for cooking and baking.

- **Sucralose**: Marketed as Splenda, sucralose is derived from sugar but is non-caloric because it is not metabolized by the body. It is heat-stable and widely used in a variety of food and beverage products.

- **Saccharin**: Sold under brand names such as Sweet'N Low, saccharin is one of the oldest artificial sweeteners. It is heat-stable and commonly used in tabletop sweeteners, diet sodas, and other low-calorie foods.

- **Acesulfame Potassium (Ace-K)**: Often combined with other artificial sweeteners to enhance sweetness, Ace-K is heat-stable and used in a variety of sugar-free products.

Artificial sweeteners are considered safe for most people when consumed in moderation as part of a balanced diet. However, some individuals may experience adverse reactions or side effects, such as headaches, digestive issues, or allergic reactions, when consuming artificial sweeteners. It's essential to monitor your body's response and consult with a healthcare professional if you have concerns.

2. Sugar Alcohols

Sugar alcohols are naturally occurring compounds found in fruits and vegetables or produced through fermentation of sugars. They provide sweetness with fewer calories than sugar and have minimal impact on blood sugar levels. Some common sugar alcohols include:

- **Erythritol**: Erythritol is a sugar alcohol with virtually no calories and a glycemic index (GI) of zero. It is well-tolerated by most people and does not cause digestive issues or tooth decay in the same way as other sugar alcohols.

- **Xylitol**: Xylitol is commonly used as a sweetener in sugar-free gum, mints, and dental products due to its ability to inhibit bacterial growth and promote dental health. However, consuming large amounts of xylitol can cause digestive discomfort and diarrhea in some individuals.

- **Sorbitol, Mannitol, and Isomalt**: These sugar alcohols are often used as sweeteners in sugar-free candies, chocolates, and baked goods. While they provide sweetness with fewer calories than sugar, they can cause gastrointestinal side effects such as gas, bloating, and diarrhea when consumed in large amounts.

Sugar alcohols are generally safe for people with diabetes when consumed in moderation. However, it's essential to be mindful of portion sizes and monitor your blood sugar levels to assess how different sugar alcohols affect your individual metabolism.

3. Natural Sweeteners

Natural sweeteners are derived from plants or natural sources and are often perceived as healthier alternatives to artificial sweeteners and sugar alcohols. While they still contain calories and carbohydrates, natural sweeteners may offer additional nutritional benefits such as vitamins, minerals, and antioxidants. Some common natural sweeteners include:

- **Stevia**: Stevia is a natural sweetener extracted from the leaves of the Stevia rebaudiana plant. It is calorie-free and has a glycemic index of zero, making it an excellent option for people with diabetes. Stevia is much sweeter than sugar, so only a small amount is needed to achieve the desired sweetness.

- **Monk Fruit Extract**: Monk fruit extract, also known as luohanguo, is derived from the monk fruit (Siraitiagrosvenorii) native to Southeast Asia. It is calorie-free and does not raise blood sugar levels, making it suitable for individuals with diabetes. Monk fruit extract is often used as a tabletop sweetener and ingredient in sugar-free products.

- **Raw Honey**: Raw honey is a natural sweetener produced by bees from the nectar of flowers. While it contains calories and carbohydrates, raw honey also provides antioxidants, enzymes, and trace minerals. It has a lower glycemic index than refined sugar, but it can still affect blood sugar levels and should be consumed in moderation by people with diabetes.

When choosing sugar substitutes and sweeteners, it's essential to consider their impact on blood sugar levels, overall health effects, and individual preferences. Experiment with different options to find the ones that work best for you and incorporate them into your diet in moderation as part of a balanced meal plan.

CHAPTER THREE

Breakfasts to Fuel Your Day

Quick and Healthy Breakfast Options for Busy Mornings

Breakfast is often hailed as the most important meal of the day, but busy mornings can make it challenging to prepare a nutritious meal. However, with a little planning and creativity, you can enjoy quick and healthy breakfast options that provide the energy and nutrients you need to start your day right. Here are some ideas for quick and healthy breakfasts for busy mornings:

1. **Overnight Oats**: Prepare a batch of overnight oats the night before by combining rolled oats with milk or yogurt, chia seeds, and your favorite toppings such as berries, nuts, seeds, or nut butter. Let the mixture soak in the refrigerator overnight, and enjoy a nutritious and filling breakfast in the morning without any cooking required.

2. **Greek Yogurt Parfait**: Layer Greek yogurt with fresh or frozen berries, sliced bananas, and a sprinkle of granola or crushed nuts for a quick and satisfying breakfast parfait. Greek yogurt is rich in protein, which helps keep you full and satisfied until your next meal.

3. **Whole Grain Toast with Nut Butter**: Toast a slice of whole grain bread and top it with your favorite nut butter (such as

almond butter or peanut butter) for a quick and portable breakfast option. Add sliced fruit or a drizzle of honey for extra flavor and nutrients.

4. **Egg Muffins**: Make a batch of egg muffins ahead of time by whisking together eggs, diced vegetables, and shredded cheese, then pouring the mixture into muffin tins and baking until set. Store the egg muffins in the refrigerator or freezer, and reheat them in the microwave for a protein-packed breakfast on the go.

5. **Smoothie Packs**: Prepare smoothie packs by portioning out frozen fruits, leafy greens, and protein powder into individual bags or containers and storing them in the freezer. In the morning, simply blend the contents of a smoothie pack with your choice of liquid (such as milk or almond milk) for a quick and nutritious breakfast smoothie.

6. **Whole Grain Cereal with Milk**: Choose a high-fiber, low-sugar cereal made from whole grains and pair it with milk or a dairy-free alternative for a simple and convenient breakfast option. Add fresh fruit or nuts for extra flavor, texture, and nutrients.

7. **Avocado Toast**: Mash half an avocado onto a slice of whole grain toast and season it with salt, pepper, and a drizzle of olive oil for a quick and satisfying breakfast. Add sliced

tomatoes, a sprinkle of feta cheese, or a poached egg for extra flavor and nutrition.

8. **Protein Pancakes or Waffles**: Make a batch of protein pancakes or waffles using a mix made with whole grain flour, protein powder, and eggs. Top them with Greek yogurt, fruit, or a drizzle of maple syrup for a nutritious and indulgent breakfast treat.

By keeping a few simple ingredients on hand and prepping ahead when possible, you can enjoy a nutritious breakfast even on the busiest of mornings. Experiment with different flavor combinations and find the breakfast options that work best for your taste preferences and lifestyle.

High-Fiber Breakfasts to Keep Blood Sugar Stable

Fiber is an essential nutrient that plays a key role in regulating blood sugar levels, promoting digestive health, and supporting overall well-being. Including high-fiber foods in your breakfast can help keep you full and satisfied, stabilize blood sugar levels, and prevent energy crashes later in the day. Here are some high-fiber breakfast ideas to incorporate into your morning routine:

1. **Oatmeal with Fruit and Nuts**: Start your day with a bowl of oatmeal made with old-fashioned rolled oats, water or milk, and a variety of toppings such as fresh or dried fruit,

chopped nuts, seeds, and a drizzle of honey or maple syrup. Oats are rich in soluble fiber, which helps slow down digestion and stabilize blood sugar levels.

2. **Chia Seed Pudding**: Make chia seed pudding by mixing chia seeds with milk or a dairy-free alternative and allowing the mixture to thicken in the refrigerator overnight. Stir in your favorite toppings such as berries, sliced bananas, shredded coconut, and a sprinkle of cinnamon for added flavor and fiber.

3. **Whole Grain Toast with Avocado and Egg**: Top a slice of whole grain toast with mashed avocado, sliced hard-boiled egg, and a sprinkle of red pepper flakes for a savory and satisfying breakfast option. The combination of fiber-rich whole grains, healthy fats from avocado, and protein from the egg helps keep you full and energized.

4. **Green Smoothie Bowl**: Blend together leafy greens such as spinach or kale, frozen fruit, Greek yogurt or silken tofu, and a splash of milk or almond milk to create a nutrient-packed green smoothie bowl. Top it with additional fruits, nuts, seeds, and granola for added fiber and texture.

5. **Whole Grain Breakfast Burrito**: Fill a whole grain tortilla with scrambled eggs or tofu, black beans, diced vegetables, salsa, and a sprinkle of cheese for a hearty and fiber-rich

breakfast burrito. Wrap it up and enjoy it on the go or as a leisurely weekend brunch option.

6. **Quinoa Breakfast Bowl**: Cook quinoa according to package instructions and serve it warm or cold with your choice of toppings such as sliced fruit, nuts, seeds, coconut flakes, and a drizzle of honey or maple syrup. Quinoa is a complete protein and a good source of fiber, making it a nutritious alternative to traditional breakfast grains.

7. **Bran Muffins**: Bake a batch of homemade bran muffins using whole grain flour, wheat bran, yogurt or applesauce, and a touch of honey or molasses for sweetness. Enjoy them warm from the oven or freeze them individually for a convenient grab-and-go breakfast option.

8. **Fruit and Yogurt Parfait**: Layer Greek yogurt with sliced fruit, granola, and a drizzle of honey or agave nectar for a simple and satisfying breakfast parfait. Greek yogurt is high in protein and low in sugar, while fruit and granola provide fiber and essential nutrients.

Incorporating high-fiber foods into your breakfast can help promote satiety, stabilize blood sugar levels, and support overall health and well-being. Experiment with different ingredients and flavor combinations to create delicious and nutritious breakfasts that fuel your day.

Diabetic-Friendly Smoothies and Breakfast Casseroles

Smoothies and breakfast casseroles are convenient and versatile options for busy mornings or leisurely weekend brunches. With the right ingredients and flavor combinations, you can create diabetic-friendly versions that provide balanced nutrition, stabilize blood sugar levels, and satisfy your taste buds. Here are some ideas for diabetic-friendly smoothies and breakfast casseroles to try:

Diabetic-Friendly Smoothies

1. **Berry Blast Smoothie**: Blend together frozen mixed berries, spinach or kale, Greek yogurt, unsweetened almond milk, and a scoop of protein powder for a nutrient-packed smoothie that's rich in fiber, vitamins, and antioxidants. Add a splash of lemon juice or a sprinkle of stevia for extra sweetness if desired.

2. **Green Power Smoothie**: Combine spinach, cucumber, avocado, banana, unsweetened almond milk, and a scoop of protein powder in a blender for a refreshing and energizing green smoothie. The combination of leafy greens, healthy fats, and protein helps keep blood sugar levels stable and promotes satiety.

3. **Peanut Butter Banana Smoothie**: Blend together ripe bananas, natural peanut butter, Greek yogurt, unsweetened almond milk, and a dash of cinnamon for a creamy and satisfying smoothie that tastes like a decadent dessert. Peanut butter provides protein and healthy fats, while bananas add natural sweetness and potassium.

4. **Chocolate Almond Smoothie**: Mix unsweetened cocoa powder, almond butter, spinach, Greek yogurt, unsweetened almond milk, and a scoop of protein powder in a blender for a rich and indulgent chocolate smoothie. The combination of cocoa powder and almond butter provides antioxidants, while spinach adds fiber and nutrients.

5. **Tropical Paradise Smoothie**: Blend together frozen pineapple, mango, banana, coconut milk or coconut water, Greek yogurt, and a scoop of protein powder for a tropical-inspired smoothie that's perfect for breakfast or post-workout recovery. Pineapple and mango provide natural sweetness and vitamin C, while coconut adds flavor and healthy fats.

Diabetic-Friendly Breakfast Casseroles

1. **Vegetable and Egg Casserole**: Whisk together eggs, egg whites, diced vegetables (such as bell peppers, onions, spinach, and mushrooms), shredded cheese, and seasonings in a baking dish. Bake until set and golden brown for a

protein-packed breakfast casserole that's loaded with fiber and nutrients.

2. **Quinoa Breakfast Casserole**: Cook quinoa according to package instructions and mix it with eggs, diced vegetables, black beans, shredded cheese, and spices in a baking dish. Bake until bubbly and golden brown for a hearty and satisfying breakfast casserole that's gluten-free and high in protein.

3. **Spinach and Feta Breakfast Strata**: Layer whole grain bread cubes, cooked spinach, crumbled feta cheese, and beaten eggs in a baking dish. Let the mixture sit in the refrigerator overnight, then bake it in the morning until puffed and golden brown for a flavorful and nutritious breakfast strata.

4. **Sweet Potato and Sausage Breakfast Bake**: Roast diced sweet potatoes until tender and mix them with cooked turkey sausage, beaten eggs, diced onions, and shredded cheese in a baking dish. Bake until set and bubbly for a hearty and satisfying breakfast bake that's packed with protein and fiber.

5. **Mexican Breakfast Casserole**: Layer corn tortillas, black beans, diced tomatoes, green chilies, scrambled eggs, and shredded cheese in a baking dish. Bake until bubbly and golden brown, then top it with avocado, salsa, and cilantro

for a flavorful and festive breakfast casserole that's sure to please.

By incorporating diabetic-friendly smoothies and breakfast casseroles into your meal rotation, you can enjoy delicious and nutritious breakfast options that support your health goals and keep you fueled throughout the day. Experiment with different ingredients, flavors, and recipes to find the combinations that work best for your taste preferences and dietary needs.

CHAPTER FOUR

Wholesome and Satisfying Lunches

Simple Salad and Wrap Recipes for Balanced Lunches

Salads and wraps are versatile and convenient options for wholesome and satisfying lunches that can be customized to suit your taste preferences and dietary needs. By combining a variety of colorful vegetables, lean proteins, healthy fats, and flavorful dressings, you can create delicious and balanced meals that keep you fueled throughout the day. Here are some simple salad and wrap recipes to try:

Salad Recipes:

1. **Greek Salad**: Toss together chopped romaine lettuce, cucumber, cherry tomatoes, red onion, Kalamata olives, and crumbled feta cheese in a large bowl. Drizzle with a mixture of olive oil, lemon juice, garlic, oregano, salt, and pepper for a classic Greek salad that's light, refreshing, and packed with flavor.

2. **Quinoa Salad**: Combine cooked quinoa with diced bell peppers, cucumbers, cherry tomatoes, red onion, black beans, corn, and avocado in a large bowl. Dress the salad with a tangy vinaigrette made from olive oil, lime juice,

cumin, chili powder, salt, and pepper for a nutritious and satisfying meal that's perfect for lunch or dinner.

3. **Asian-Inspired Salad**: Mix together shredded cabbage, carrots, bell peppers, snap peas, edamame, and sliced almonds in a large bowl. Toss the salad with a sesame ginger dressing made from soy sauce, rice vinegar, sesame oil, ginger, garlic, honey, and sriracha for a flavorful and colorful salad that's full of crunch and texture.

4. **Mediterranean Chickpea Salad**: Combine cooked chickpeas with diced cucumber, cherry tomatoes, red onion, bell pepper, parsley, and feta cheese in a large bowl. Dress the salad with a lemon herb vinaigrette made from olive oil, lemon juice, garlic, oregano, salt, and pepper for a protein-rich and satisfying salad that's bursting with Mediterranean flavors.

Wrap Recipes:

1. **Grilled Veggie Wrap**: Fill a whole grain tortilla with grilled vegetables such as zucchini, bell peppers, eggplant, and onions. Add a smear of hummus or tzatziki sauce for creaminess, and sprinkle with crumbled feta cheese or sliced olives for extra flavor. Roll up the wrap tightly and enjoy it as a nutritious and portable lunch option.

2. **Turkey and Avocado Wrap**: Layer thinly sliced turkey breast, avocado, lettuce, tomato, cucumber, and shredded carrots on a whole grain tortilla. Drizzle with a squeeze of lemon juice or a dollop of Greek yogurt for added moisture and flavor. Roll up the wrap tightly and secure it with toothpicks for a protein-packed and satisfying lunch.

3. **Asian Chicken Wrap**: Fill a whole grain tortilla with cooked shredded chicken breast, shredded cabbage, shredded carrots, sliced bell peppers, and chopped cilantro. Drizzle with a homemade peanut sauce made from peanut butter, soy sauce, rice vinegar, honey, garlic, and ginger for a savory and satisfying wrap with an Asian twist.

4. **Tuna Salad Wrap**: Mix together canned tuna, Greek yogurt, diced celery, diced red onion, chopped pickles, and a squeeze of lemon juice in a bowl. Spread the tuna salad onto a whole grain tortilla, top with lettuce leaves, and roll up tightly for a protein-rich and flavorful wrap that's perfect for lunch on the go.

By incorporating simple salad and wrap recipes into your meal rotation, you can enjoy wholesome and satisfying lunches that provide the nutrients you need to stay fueled and energized throughout the day. Experiment with different ingredients, flavors, and dressings to create delicious and balanced meals that suit your taste preferences and dietary goals.

Protein-Packed Lunches to Keep You Full and Energized

Protein is an essential nutrient that plays a key role in supporting muscle growth and repair, stabilizing blood sugar levels, and promoting feelings of fullness and satiety. Including protein-rich foods in your lunch can help keep you fueled and energized throughout the day, preventing mid-afternoon energy crashes and cravings. Here are some protein-packed lunch ideas to try:

1. **Grilled Chicken Salad**: Start with a base of mixed greens or spinach and top it with grilled chicken breast, sliced avocado, cherry tomatoes, cucumbers, and shredded carrots. Drizzle the salad with a light vinaigrette or Greek yogurt dressing for added flavor and enjoy a nutritious and satisfying lunch that's high in protein and low in carbs.

2. **Quinoa and Black Bean Bowl**: Combine cooked quinoa with black beans, diced bell peppers, corn, cherry tomatoes, avocado, and cilantro in a bowl. Drizzle the bowl with a lime cilantro dressing made from olive oil, lime juice, garlic, cilantro, salt, and pepper for a protein-packed and flavorful lunch that's vegetarian-friendly and gluten-free.

3. **Salmon and Quinoa Salad**: Flake cooked salmon over a bed of mixed greens or spinach and top it with cooked quinoa, sliced cucumber, cherry tomatoes, red onion, and feta cheese. Drizzle the salad with a lemon herb vinaigrette or

tzatziki sauce for a protein-rich and satisfying lunch that's rich in omega-3 fatty acids and essential nutrients.

4. **Egg Salad Wrap**: Mix together hard-boiled eggs, Greek yogurt, diced celery, diced red onion, chopped pickles, and a squeeze of lemon juice in a bowl. Spread the egg salad onto a whole grain tortilla, top with lettuce leaves, and roll up tightly for a protein-packed and portable lunch option that's perfect for on the go.

5. **Tofu Stir-Fry with Brown Rice**: Stir-fry cubed tofu with mixed vegetables such as bell peppers, broccoli, carrots, and snap peas in a skillet with a splash of soy sauce and sesame oil. Serve the tofu stir-fry over cooked brown rice for a protein-rich and satisfying lunch that's packed with flavor and nutrients.

6. **Turkey and Veggie Lettuce Wraps**: Fill large lettuce leaves with sliced turkey breast, sliced avocado, shredded carrots, cucumber slices, and hummus or tzatziki sauce. Roll up the lettuce leaves and secure them with toothpicks for a low-carb and protein-packed lunch option that's light, refreshing, and portable.

7. **Chickpea and Spinach Salad**: Toss together cooked chickpeas with baby spinach, diced cucumber, cherry tomatoes, red onion, and feta cheese in a bowl. Dress the salad with a lemon herb vinaigrette or balsamic vinaigrette

for a protein-rich and fiber-packed lunch that's vegetarian-friendly and full of flavor.

8. **Shrimp and Avocado Salad**: Combine cooked shrimp with sliced avocado, mixed greens, cherry tomatoes, cucumber slices, and sliced bell peppers in a bowl. Drizzle the salad with a cilantro lime dressing or creamy avocado dressing for a protein-packed and refreshing lunch that's perfect for warm weather.

By incorporating protein-rich foods into your lunch, you can stay full and satisfied throughout the day while supporting your overall health and well-being. Experiment with different protein sources, flavor combinations, and meal prep techniques to create delicious and nutritious lunches that suit your taste preferences and lifestyle.

Creative Lunch Ideas for Work or School

Coming up with creative and satisfying lunch ideas for work or school can help break up the monotony of mealtime and keep you excited about your midday meal. Whether you're packing a lunchbox to take with you or preparing a meal to enjoy at home, thinking outside the box can lead to delicious and nutritious lunches that satisfy your taste buds and fuel your body. Here are some creative lunch ideas to try:

1. **Bento Box Lunch**: Pack a bento box or divided container with a variety of bite-sized snacks and mini meals for a fun and

interactive lunch experience. Include items such as sliced vegetables with hummus, cheese and crackers, fruit skewers, hard-boiled eggs, and mini sandwiches for a balanced and satisfying meal on the go.

2. **DIY Salad Bar**: Set up a DIY salad bar at home or work with a selection of fresh greens, chopped vegetables, cooked proteins, grains, nuts, seeds, and dressings. Allow everyone to customize their own salad creation according to their taste preferences and dietary needs for a fun and interactive lunch experience that's sure to please.

3. **Soup and Sandwich Combo**: Pair a hearty soup with a grilled cheese sandwich or wrap for a comforting and satisfying lunch that's perfect for cooler weather. Choose soups such as tomato basil, butternut squash, lentil, or minestrone and pair them with a sandwich or wrap filled with your favorite fillings for a balanced and satisfying meal.

4. **DIY Sushi Rolls**: Roll up your own sushi rolls at home using nori seaweed sheets, sushi rice, sliced vegetables, avocado, cooked shrimp or tofu, and your favorite condiments such as soy sauce, wasabi, and pickled ginger. Get creative with different fillings and flavor combinations to create delicious and nutritious sushi rolls that are perfect for lunch or a snack.

5. **Mason Jar Salads**: Layer ingredients for a salad in a mason jar starting with dressing on the bottom, followed by hearty vegetables, grains, proteins, and greens on top. Seal the jar and refrigerate until ready to eat, then shake it up and enjoy a fresh and flavorful salad that stays crisp and delicious until lunchtime.

6. **Stuffed Pita Pockets**: Fill whole wheat pita pockets with a variety of fillings such as grilled chicken, falafel, hummus, tabbouleh, shredded lettuce, diced tomatoes, and sliced cucumbers for a portable and satisfying lunch option that's perfect for eating on the go.

7. **Build-Your-Own Taco Bar**: Set up a build-your-own taco bar with a selection of taco shells or tortillas, cooked proteins such as grilled chicken, beef, or fish, shredded cheese, lettuce, tomato, salsa, guacamole, and sour cream. Allow everyone to assemble their own tacos according to their taste preferences for a fun and customizable lunch experience.

8. **Savory Breakfast for Lunch**: Enjoy breakfast for lunch by whipping up savory dishes such as omelets, frittatas, breakfast burritos, or egg muffins filled with vegetables, cheese, and protein. Serve them with a side of whole grain toast, fresh fruit, or a mixed green salad for a balanced and satisfying midday meal.

By thinking creatively and outside the box, you can come up with delicious and satisfying lunch ideas that keep mealtime exciting and enjoyable. Experiment with different ingredients, flavors, and presentation techniques to create meals that nourish your body and satisfy your taste buds, whether you're at work, school, or home.

CHAPTER FIVE

Nourishing Dinners for Every Taste

Easy One-Pot Dinners for Weeknight Convenience

One-pot dinners are a lifesaver on busy weeknights when you want to enjoy a nourishing meal without spending hours in the kitchen or dealing with a sink full of dishes. These meals are convenient, flavorful, and versatile, allowing you to customize them with your favorite ingredients and flavors. Here are some easy one-pot dinner ideas to try:

1. **Chicken and Vegetable Stir-Fry**: In a large skillet or wok, stir-fry diced chicken breast with a variety of vegetables such as bell peppers, broccoli, carrots, snap peas, and mushrooms. Season with garlic, ginger, soy sauce, and sesame oil for a quick and flavorful stir-fry that's perfect served over rice or noodles.

2. **One-Pot Pasta Primavera**: Cook pasta in a large pot of boiling water according to package instructions, adding diced vegetables such as zucchini, cherry tomatoes, asparagus, and spinach during the last few minutes of cooking. Drain the pasta and vegetables, then toss them with olive oil, garlic, fresh herbs, and grated Parmesan cheese for a simple and satisfying pasta dish.

3. **Beef and Vegetable Chili**: Brown ground beef in a large Dutch oven or slow cooker, then add diced onions, bell peppers, garlic, diced tomatoes, kidney beans, black beans, corn, chili powder, cumin, and paprika. Simmer the chili for about 30 minutes to allow the flavors to meld together, then serve it hot topped with shredded cheese, sour cream, and sliced green onions.

4. **Shrimp and Sausage Jambalaya**: In a large skillet or Dutch oven, sauté sliced sausage and diced onions, bell peppers, and celery until softened. Add diced tomatoes, rice, chicken broth, Cajun seasoning, and raw shrimp, then cover and simmer until the rice is cooked and the shrimp are pink and cooked through. Serve the jambalaya hot with a sprinkle of chopped parsley for a taste of the South.

5. **Vegetable and Bean Soup**: In a large pot, sauté diced onions, carrots, celery, and garlic until softened. Add vegetable broth, diced tomatoes, canned beans (such as cannellini beans or chickpeas), chopped kale or spinach, dried herbs, and cooked pasta or grains if desired. Simmer the soup until the vegetables are tender and the flavors have melded together, then serve it hot with crusty bread for dipping.

6. **Tofu and Vegetable Curry**: In a large skillet or saucepan, sauté diced tofu with curry paste, diced onions, bell peppers, carrots, and potatoes until the vegetables are tender. Add

coconut milk, vegetable broth, and frozen peas, then simmer until heated through and the flavors have melded together. Serve the curry hot over rice or quinoa for a flavorful and satisfying meal.

7. **Italian Sausage and Vegetable Skillet**: Brown Italian sausage in a large skillet, then add diced onions, bell peppers, zucchini, cherry tomatoes, and garlic. Sauté until the vegetables are tender and the sausage is cooked through, then season with Italian herbs, salt, and pepper. Serve the skillet hot with crusty bread or cooked pasta for a hearty and delicious dinner.

8. **Lentil and Vegetable Stew**: In a large pot or Dutch oven, sauté diced onions, carrots, celery, and garlic until softened. Add dried lentils, diced tomatoes, vegetable broth, and chopped kale or spinach, then simmer until the lentils are tender and the flavors have melded together. Serve the stew hot with a sprinkle of fresh parsley or a dollop of Greek yogurt for added flavor and creaminess.

By preparing one-pot dinners, you can enjoy delicious and nourishing meals with minimal effort and cleanup, making them perfect for busy weeknights or lazy weekends. Experiment with different ingredients, flavors, and seasonings to create customized dishes that suit your taste preferences and dietary needs.

Flavorful Vegetarian and Plant-Based Dinner Options

Vegetarian and plant-based dinners are not only delicious and satisfying but also packed with nutrients and beneficial for your health and the environment. Whether you're a committed vegetarian or simply looking to incorporate more plant-based meals into your diet, there are plenty of flavorful and satisfying options to choose from. Here are some ideas for vegetarian and plant-based dinner options:

1. **Vegetable Stir-Fry with Tofu**: Sauté diced tofu with a variety of vegetables such as bell peppers, broccoli, carrots, snap peas, and mushrooms in a large skillet or wok. Season with garlic, ginger, soy sauce, and sesame oil for a quick and flavorful stir-fry that's high in protein and fiber. Serve it over rice or noodles for a complete meal.

2. **Quinoa and Black Bean Tacos**: Cook quinoa according to package instructions and season it with taco seasoning. Fill taco shells or tortillas with seasoned quinoa, black beans, shredded lettuce, diced tomatoes, avocado slices, and a dollop of Greek yogurt or salsa for a nutritious and satisfying taco night.

3. **Eggplant Parmesan**: Slice eggplant into rounds and bread them with breadcrumbs and Parmesan cheese. Bake the breaded eggplant until golden brown and crispy, then layer it

with marinara sauce and mozzarella cheese. Bake until the cheese is melted and bubbly, then serve the eggplant Parmesan hot with a side of pasta or a green salad.

4. **Mushroom and Spinach Risotto**: Sauté diced onions and garlic in a large skillet until softened, then add Arborio rice and cook until toasted. Gradually add vegetable broth, stirring constantly, until the rice is creamy and cooked through. Stir in sautéed mushrooms, chopped spinach, Parmesan cheese, and a splash of white wine for a comforting and flavorful risotto.

5. **Chickpea and Vegetable Curry**: Sauté diced onions, bell peppers, carrots, and potatoes in a large skillet or saucepan until softened. Add canned chickpeas, diced tomatoes, coconut milk, and curry paste, then simmer until the vegetables are tender and the flavors have melded together. Serve the curry hot over rice or quinoa for a hearty and satisfying meal.

6. **Sweet Potato and Black Bean Enchiladas**: Roast diced sweet potatoes until tender, then combine them with black beans, diced onions, bell peppers, and spices such as cumin, chili powder, and garlic powder. Roll the mixture into corn tortillas, place them in a baking dish, and top them with enchilada sauce and shredded cheese. Bake until the

enchiladas are heated through and the cheese is melted and bubbly, then serve them hot with a side of rice or salad.

7. **Vegetable and Lentil Shepherd's Pie**: Sauté diced onions, carrots, celery, and garlic in a large skillet until softened, then add cooked lentils, diced tomatoes, vegetable broth, and frozen peas. Simmer until heated through and the flavors have melded together, then transfer the mixture to a baking dish. Top with mashed potatoes and bake until golden brown and bubbly for a comforting and satisfying shepherd's pie.

8. **Spinach and Ricotta Stuffed Shells**: Cook jumbo pasta shells according to package instructions, then fill them with a mixture of ricotta cheese, chopped spinach, garlic, Parmesan cheese, and herbs. Place the stuffed shells in a baking dish, top them with marinara sauce and mozzarella cheese, and bake until heated through and the cheese is melted and bubbly. Serve the stuffed shells hot with a side of garlic bread or a green salad.

By incorporating vegetarian and plant-based dinners into your meal rotation, you can enjoy delicious and nutritious meals that are good for you and the planet. Experiment with different ingredients, flavors, and cuisines to create flavorful and satisfying dishes that appeal to your taste buds and dietary preferences.

Comforting Slow Cooker and Instant Pot Recipes

Slow cookers and Instant Pots are invaluable tools for creating comforting and flavorful meals with minimal effort and hands-on time. These kitchen appliances allow you to set and forget your dinner, resulting in tender and delicious dishes that are perfect for busy weeknights or lazy weekends. Here are some comforting slow cooker and Instant Pot recipes to try:

Slow Cooker Recipes:

1. **Beef Stew**: Combine cubed beef chuck roast with diced onions, carrots, celery, potatoes, and garlic in a slow cooker. Season with salt, pepper, thyme, rosemary, and bay leaves, then add beef broth and tomato paste. Cook on low for 8 hours or until the beef is tender and the vegetables are cooked through. Serve the beef stew hot with crusty bread for dipping.

2. **Chicken Tikka Masala**: Place chicken thighs, diced onions, bell peppers, garlic, ginger, diced tomatoes, coconut milk, and Tikka Masala seasoning in a slow cooker. Cook on low for 6 hours or until the chicken is cooked through and the flavors have melded together. Serve the Chicken Tikka Masala hot over rice with naan bread for a flavorful and satisfying meal.

3. **Pulled Pork Sandwiches**: Rub a pork shoulder with a mixture of brown sugar, paprika, garlic powder, onion powder, salt, and pepper, then place it in a slow cooker. Add diced onions, apple cider vinegar, and chicken broth, then cook on low for 8 hours or until the pork is tender and falls apart easily. Shred the pork with two forks and serve it on buns with barbecue sauce and coleslaw for a classic pulled pork sandwich.

4. **Vegetarian Chili**: Combine diced onions, bell peppers, carrots, celery, garlic, diced tomatoes, kidney beans, black beans, corn, chili powder, cumin, and paprika in a slow cooker. Cook on low for 6 hours or until the vegetables are tender and the flavors have melded together. Serve the vegetarian chili hot with shredded cheese, sour cream, and sliced green onions for a hearty and satisfying meal.

5. **Lentil Soup**: Sauté diced onions, carrots, celery, and garlic in a skillet until softened, then transfer them to a slow cooker. Add dried lentils, diced tomatoes, vegetable broth, bay leaves, and dried herbs such as thyme and rosemary. Cook on low for 8 hours or until the lentils are tender and the flavors have melded together. Serve the lentil soup hot with crusty bread for dipping.

6. **Pot Roast**: Place a beef chuck roast in a slow cooker and season it with salt, pepper, garlic powder, and onion

powder. Add diced onions, carrots, celery, potatoes, and garlic, then pour beef broth and Worcestershire sauce over the top. Cook on low for 8 hours or until the beef is tender and falls apart easily. Serve the pot roast hot with mashed potatoes and roasted vegetables for a comforting and satisfying meal.

7. **Coconut Curry Chicken**: Place chicken thighs, diced onions, bell peppers, carrots, potatoes, garlic, ginger, coconut milk, curry powder, and a splash of lime juice in a slow cooker. Cook on low for 6 hours or until the chicken is cooked through and the vegetables are tender. Serve the coconut curry chicken hot over rice with naan bread for a flavorful and satisfying meal.

8. **Buffalo Chicken Dip**: Combine shredded chicken breast, cream cheese, shredded cheddar cheese, buffalo sauce, and ranch dressing mix in a slow cooker. Cook on low for 2-3 hours or until the dip is hot and bubbly, stirring occasionally. Serve the buffalo chicken dip hot with tortilla chips, celery sticks, and carrot sticks for a crowd-pleasing appetizer or game day snack.

By using slow cookers and Instant Pots, you can create comforting and flavorful meals with minimal effort and hands-on time. Experiment with different ingredients, flavors, and cooking techniques to create delicious and satisfying dishes that are perfect for busy weeknights or lazy weekends.

CHAPTER SIX

Smart Snacking Strategies

Nutrient-Dense Snack Ideas for Between Meals

Smart snacking is an essential part of maintaining energy levels and managing hunger throughout the day. Choosing nutrient-dense snacks that provide a balance of macronutrients (carbohydrates, protein, and fats) can help keep you satisfied and fueled until your next meal. Here are some nutrient-dense snack ideas to try:

1. **Greek Yogurt with Berries**: Greek yogurt is high in protein and calcium, making it a satisfying and nutritious snack. Top a serving of Greek yogurt with fresh berries such as strawberries, blueberries, or raspberries for added fiber, antioxidants, and natural sweetness.

2. **Apple Slices with Nut Butter**: Apples are rich in fiber and vitamin C, while nut butter provides healthy fats and protein. Spread almond butter, peanut butter, or cashew butter onto apple slices for a crunchy and satisfying snack that's perfect for on-the-go.

3. **Hard-Boiled Eggs**: Eggs are an excellent source of high-quality protein and essential nutrients such as vitamin D and choline. Keep a batch of hard-boiled eggs in the fridge for a

quick and easy snack option that provides long-lasting energy and satiety.

4. **Mixed Nuts and Dried Fruit**: Nuts and dried fruit are a convenient and portable snack option that provides a balance of healthy fats, protein, and carbohydrates. Mix together almonds, walnuts, cashews, or pistachios with dried cranberries, apricots, or raisins for a satisfying and energizing snack.

5. **Hummus and Veggie Sticks**: Hummus is made from chickpeas, which are rich in protein and fiber, while raw vegetables such as carrot sticks, cucumber slices, and bell pepper strips provide vitamins, minerals, and antioxidants. Dip veggie sticks into hummus for a crunchy and nutritious snack that's perfect for satisfying midday hunger.

6. **Cottage Cheese with Cherry Tomatoes**: Cottage cheese is a rich source of protein and calcium, while cherry tomatoes provide vitamin C and antioxidants. Top a serving of cottage cheese with halved cherry tomatoes and a sprinkle of black pepper for a refreshing and satisfying snack option.

7. **Whole Grain Crackers with Avocado**: Whole grain crackers are a good source of fiber and complex carbohydrates, while avocado provides healthy fats and essential nutrients such as potassium and vitamin E. Spread mashed avocado onto

whole grain crackers for a delicious and filling snack that's rich in flavor and nutrients.

8. **Edamame**: Edamame, or young soybeans, are a nutritious and protein-rich snack that's packed with essential amino acids, fiber, and vitamins. Enjoy steamed edamame sprinkled with sea salt for a satisfying and savory snack that's perfect for munching on between meals.

By choosing nutrient-dense snacks that provide a balance of macronutrients and essential nutrients, you can keep hunger at bay and maintain energy levels throughout the day. Experiment with different combinations of foods and flavors to find snack options that suit your taste preferences and dietary needs.

Homemade Snacks That Are Low in Sugar and High in Flavor

When it comes to snacking, homemade options are often the healthiest choice because they allow you to control the ingredients and avoid added sugars, artificial flavors, and preservatives. By making your own snacks at home, you can create delicious and nutritious options that are low in sugar and high in flavor. Here are some homemade snack ideas to try:

1. **Homemade Trail Mix**: Combine unsalted nuts such as almonds, cashews, and walnuts with unsweetened dried fruit such as raisins, cranberries, and apricots. Add a sprinkle

of dark chocolate chips or cacao nibs for a touch of sweetness and indulgence. Portion out the trail mix into individual servings for a convenient grab-and-go snack option.

2. **Baked Veggie Chips**: Slice vegetables such as sweet potatoes, beets, zucchini, or kale into thin slices, then toss them with olive oil and your favorite seasonings such as sea salt, black pepper, garlic powder, or smoked paprika. Arrange the seasoned vegetable slices in a single layer on a baking sheet and bake them at a low temperature until crispy and golden brown. Enjoy the baked veggie chips as a crunchy and flavorful snack that's perfect for satisfying salty cravings.

3. **Homemade Granola Bars**: Make your own granola bars using rolled oats, nuts, seeds, dried fruit, and natural sweeteners such as honey, maple syrup, or dates. Mix together the ingredients in a bowl, press the mixture into a lined baking dish, and bake until golden brown and firm. Once cooled, cut the granola mixture into bars or squares for a wholesome and satisfying snack that's perfect for on-the-go.

4. **Roasted Chickpeas**: Drain and rinse canned chickpeas, then toss them with olive oil and your favorite seasonings such as smoked paprika, cumin, chili powder, or garlic powder. Spread the seasoned chickpeas in a single layer on a baking

sheet and roast them in the oven until crispy and golden brown. Enjoy the roasted chickpeas as a crunchy and protein-rich snack that's perfect for munching on between meals.

5. **Homemade Fruit Leather**: Puree fresh or frozen fruit such as strawberries, raspberries, mangoes, or apples in a blender until smooth. Spread the fruit puree in a thin layer onto a lined baking sheet and bake it at a low temperature until set and slightly tacky. Once cooled, cut the fruit leather into strips or shapes for a natural and flavorful snack that's free of added sugars and artificial ingredients.

6. **Energy Bites**: Combine rolled oats, nut butter, honey or maple syrup, and mix-ins such as chia seeds, flaxseeds, shredded coconut, or dark chocolate chips in a bowl. Roll the mixture into bite-sized balls and refrigerate them until firm. Enjoy the energy bites as a convenient and portable snack that's packed with protein, fiber, and natural sweetness.

7. **Homemade Popcorn**: Air-pop popcorn kernels using a popcorn maker or stovetop popper, then toss the popcorn with melted coconut oil or olive oil and your favorite seasonings such as nutritional yeast, sea salt, garlic powder, or dried herbs. Enjoy the homemade popcorn as a light and crunchy snack that's perfect for satisfying salty cravings without the added butter or artificial flavors.

8. **Chia Seed Pudding**: Mix together chia seeds, almond milk or coconut milk, and natural sweeteners such as maple syrup or honey in a jar or bowl. Stir well to combine, then refrigerate the mixture for several hours or overnight until thickened. Once set, top the chia seed pudding with fresh fruit, nuts, or seeds for a nutritious and satisfying snack that's rich in fiber and omega-3 fatty acids.

By making your own snacks at home, you can enjoy delicious and nutritious options that are low in sugar and high in flavor. Experiment with different ingredients, flavors, and recipes to create homemade snacks that suit your taste preferences and dietary needs.

Portable Snacks for On-the-Go Convenience

When you're on the go, having portable snacks on hand can help keep hunger at bay and prevent unhealthy food choices. Portable snacks are convenient, easy to transport, and can be enjoyed anywhere, whether you're traveling, running errands, or at work or school. Here are some portable snack ideas to try:

1. **Nut and Seed Bars**: Choose nut and seed bars made with wholesome ingredients such as nuts, seeds, dried fruit, and natural sweeteners. Look for options that are low in added sugars and free of artificial flavors and preservatives for a nutritious and satisfying snack that's perfect for on-the-go.

2. **String Cheese**: String cheese is a convenient and portable snack option that provides protein, calcium, and essential nutrients. Pack individually wrapped string cheese sticks in your bag or lunchbox for a quick and easy snack that's perfect for satisfying midday hunger.

3. **Whole Fruit**: Whole fruits such as apples, bananas, oranges, and grapes are naturally portable and require no preparation. Pack a piece of fruit in your bag or purse for a nutritious and refreshing snack that's rich in vitamins, minerals, and fiber.

4. **Individual Packs of Nuts**: Opt for individual packs of nuts such as almonds, walnuts, or pistachios for a convenient and portion-controlled snack option. Nuts are rich in healthy fats, protein, and fiber, making them a satisfying and energizing snack that's perfect for on-the-go.

5. **Rice Cakes with Nut Butter**: Spread nut butter such as almond butter or peanut butter onto rice cakes for a portable and satisfying snack that's perfect for on-the-go. Pack the rice cakes in a small container or resealable bag for easy transport and enjoy them anytime, anywhere.

6. **Dried Fruit**: Dried fruit such as apricots, raisins, mangoes, and cranberries are naturally sweet and portable, making them an ideal snack option for on-the-go. Pack individual servings of dried fruit in small containers or resealable bags

for a convenient and nutritious snack that's perfect for satisfying sweet cravings.

7. **Yogurt Cups**: Choose single-serve cups of yogurt for a convenient and portable snack option that's rich in protein and probiotics. Look for options that are low in added sugars and free of artificial flavors and preservatives for a nutritious and satisfying snack that's perfect for on-the-go.

8. **Whole Grain Crackers with Cheese**: Pack individual servings of whole grain crackers and cheese for a portable and satisfying snack that provides a balance of carbohydrates, protein, and fats. Choose whole grain crackers and natural cheese for a nutritious and flavorful snack that's perfect for on-the-go.

By having portable snacks on hand, you can stay fueled and satisfied throughout the day, even when you're on the go. Experiment with different snack options and combinations to find portable snacks that suit your taste preferences and dietary needs.

CHAPTER SEVEN

Decadent Desserts Made Diabetic-Friendly

Lower-Sugar Dessert Recipes for Satisfying Sweet Cravings

Satisfying sweet cravings while managing diabetes can be challenging, but with the right recipes and ingredients, it's possible to enjoy decadent desserts without causing large spikes in blood sugar levels. Lower-sugar dessert recipes focus on reducing added sugars while still providing delicious flavors and textures. Here are some lower-sugar dessert ideas to try:

1. **Dark Chocolate-Dipped Strawberries**: Dip fresh strawberries in melted dark chocolate that's at least 70% cocoa for a decadent and satisfying treat. Dark chocolate contains less sugar than milk chocolate and provides antioxidants, making it a healthier option for satisfying sweet cravings.

2. **Baked Apples with Cinnamon**: Core and slice apples, then sprinkle them with cinnamon and a touch of natural sweetener such as stevia or monk fruit sweetener. Bake the apples until tender and caramelized for a warm and comforting dessert that's perfect for cooler evenings.

3. **Greek Yogurt Parfait**: Layer Greek yogurt with fresh berries, sliced almonds, and a drizzle of honey or maple syrup for a creamy and satisfying dessert option that's high in protein

and lower in added sugars. Customize the parfait with your favorite fruits and toppings for endless flavor variations.

4. **Chia Seed Pudding**: Mix chia seeds with unsweetened almond milk or coconut milk, vanilla extract, and a touch of natural sweetener such as agave syrup or erythritol. Let the mixture sit in the refrigerator until thickened, then top it with fresh fruit, nuts, or seeds for a nutritious and satisfying dessert that's rich in fiber and omega-3 fatty acids.

5. **No-Bake Energy Bites**: Combine rolled oats, nut butter, chopped nuts, seeds, dried fruit, and a touch of honey or maple syrup in a bowl. Roll the mixture into bite-sized balls and refrigerate until firm. Enjoy the energy bites as a satisfying and portable dessert option that's perfect for curbing sweet cravings.

6. **Coconut Macaroons**: Mix shredded coconut with egg whites, vanilla extract, and a touch of natural sweetener such as stevia or erythritol. Form the mixture into small mounds and bake until golden brown and crisp. Enjoy the coconut macaroons as a sweet and satisfying dessert that's lower in sugar and carbohydrates.

7. **Frozen Banana Bites**: Slice bananas into rounds and spread peanut butter or almond butter between two slices to create sandwiches. Dip the banana sandwiches in melted dark

chocolate and freeze until firm for a delicious and satisfying frozen treat that's perfect for satisfying sweet cravings.

8. **Almond Flour Brownies**: Use almond flour or coconut flour instead of traditional flour to make brownies that are lower in carbohydrates and higher in fiber and protein. Sweeten the brownies with natural sweeteners such as stevia, erythritol, or monk fruit sweetener for a decadent and satisfying dessert option that's perfect for indulging in without guilt.

By using lower-sugar dessert recipes and natural sweeteners, you can enjoy satisfying sweet cravings while managing your blood sugar levels. Experiment with different ingredients and flavor combinations to create delicious and indulgent desserts that fit into your diabetic-friendly diet.

Fruit-Based Desserts That Are Naturally Sweet and Healthy

Fruit-based desserts are naturally sweet and packed with vitamins, minerals, and antioxidants, making them a healthier option for satisfying sweet cravings while managing diabetes. By incorporating fresh or frozen fruit into dessert recipes, you can create delicious and nutritious treats that are lower in added sugars and higher in fiber. Here are some fruit-based dessert ideas to try:

1. **Grilled Pineapple with Coconut Yogurt**: Grill pineapple slices until caramelized and golden brown, then serve them with a dollop of coconut yogurt and a sprinkle of shredded coconut for a tropical and refreshing dessert that's perfect for summer.

2. **Mixed Berry Crisp**: Toss together fresh or frozen berries such as strawberries, blueberries, and raspberries with a touch of natural sweetener such as stevia or monk fruit sweetener. Top the berry mixture with a crumbly topping made from oats, almond flour, coconut oil, and cinnamon, then bake until golden brown and bubbly for a warm and comforting dessert.

3. **Banana Nice Cream**: Blend frozen bananas with a splash of almond milk or coconut milk until smooth and creamy, then add flavorings such as vanilla extract, cocoa powder, or peanut butter for extra indulgence. Enjoy the banana nice cream as a guilt-free and refreshing dessert option that's perfect for satisfying sweet cravings.

4. **Baked Pears with Cinnamon**: Core and halve pears, then sprinkle them with cinnamon and a touch of natural sweetener such as honey or maple syrup. Bake the pears until tender and caramelized, then serve them warm with a scoop of Greek yogurt or a drizzle of almond butter for a simple and satisfying dessert option.

5. **Mango Coconut Sorbet**: Blend ripe mango chunks with coconut milk and a touch of lime juice until smooth and creamy, then freeze the mixture until firm. Scoop the mango coconut sorbet into bowls or cones for a refreshing and tropical dessert that's naturally sweet and full of flavor.

6. **Berry Chia Seed Jam**: Simmer mixed berries such as strawberries, raspberries, and blackberries with a touch of natural sweetener such as honey or maple syrup until soft and syrupy. Stir in chia seeds and let the mixture cool and thicken, then spread it onto whole grain toast or use it as a topping for yogurt or oatmeal for a nutritious and delicious dessert option.

7. **Apple Cinnamon Oat Bars**: Mix together diced apples, cinnamon, oats, almond flour, and a touch of natural sweetener such as stevia or monk fruit sweetener in a bowl. Press the mixture into a baking dish and bake until golden brown and crisp, then cut it into bars for a wholesome and satisfying dessert that's perfect for on-the-go.

8. **Frozen Yogurt Bark**: Spread Greek yogurt onto a baking sheet lined with parchment paper, then top it with sliced fruit such as strawberries, kiwi, and mango. Drizzle the yogurt with a touch of honey or maple syrup for sweetness, then freeze until firm. Break the frozen yogurt bark into

pieces and enjoy it as a refreshing and nutritious dessert option that's perfect for hot summer days.

By incorporating fresh or frozen fruit into dessert recipes, you can create delicious and nutritious treats that are naturally sweet and healthy. Experiment with different fruits, flavorings, and sweeteners to create fruit-based desserts that satisfy your sweet cravings while supporting your overall health and well-being.

Indulgent Treats Made Healthier with Smart Ingredient Swaps

Indulgent treats such as cookies, cakes, and desserts are often high in sugar, refined carbohydrates, and unhealthy fats, making them less than ideal for individuals with diabetes. However, by making smart ingredient swaps and modifications, you can transform traditional indulgent treats into healthier options that are lower in added sugars and higher in fiber and nutrients. Here are some indulgent treats made healthier with smart ingredient swaps:

1. **Whole Wheat Chocolate Chip Cookies**: Use whole wheat flour instead of all-purpose flour to make chocolate chip cookies that are higher in fiber and nutrients. Sweeten the cookies with natural sweeteners such as coconut sugar or maple syrup, and use dark chocolate chips that are at least 70% cocoa for a richer flavor and lower sugar content.

2. **Avocado Brownies**: Replace butter or oil with mashed avocado in brownie recipes to reduce saturated fat and increase heart-healthy monounsaturated fats. Avocado also adds creaminess and moisture to brownies, making them rich and fudgy without the need for excess fat.

3. **Almond Flour Cake**: Use almond flour or coconut flour instead of traditional flour to make cakes that are lower in carbohydrates and higher in protein and fiber. Sweeten the cake with natural sweeteners such as stevia or erythritol, and add flavorings such as vanilla extract, almond extract, or citrus zest for extra depth of flavor.

4. **Coconut Oil Granola Bars**: Substitute coconut oil for butter or margarine in granola bar recipes to reduce saturated fat and increase medium-chain triglycerides, which may have metabolic benefits for individuals with diabetes. Add nuts, seeds, dried fruit, and natural sweeteners such as honey or maple syrup for texture and sweetness.

5. **Black Bean Brownies**: Replace flour with pureed black beans in brownie recipes to boost fiber and protein content while reducing carbohydrates. Black beans also add moisture and fudginess to brownies, making them dense and satisfying without the need for excess sugar or fat.

6. **Oatmeal Raisin Cookies**: Use rolled oats instead of refined flour in oatmeal raisin cookie recipes to increase fiber

content and slow the release of sugar into the bloodstream. Sweeten the cookies with natural sweeteners such as honey or molasses, and add cinnamon and nutmeg for warm and comforting flavor.

7. **Quinoa Chocolate Cake**: Substitute cooked quinoa for flour in chocolate cake recipes to add protein, fiber, and essential nutrients such as magnesium and iron. Quinoa also adds moisture and richness to cakes, making them tender and flavorful without the need for excess sugar or fat.

8. **Chia Seed Pudding Parfaits**: Use chia seeds instead of traditional thickeners such as cornstarch or gelatin in pudding recipes to increase fiber content and add omega-3 fatty acids. Layer the chia seed pudding with fresh fruit, nuts, and seeds for a nutritious and satisfying parfait that's perfect for dessert or breakfast.

By making smart ingredient swaps and modifications, you can transform indulgent treats into healthier options that are lower in added sugars and higher in fiber and nutrients. Experiment with different ingredients, flavors, and recipes to create indulgent treats that satisfy your sweet cravings while supporting your overall health and well-being.

CHAPTER EIGHT

Flavorful Side Dishes to Complement Any Meal

Simple Vegetable Side Dishes Packed with Nutrients

Vegetable side dishes are an essential part of any meal, providing vitamins, minerals, fiber, and antioxidants to support overall health and well-being. Simple vegetable side dishes are easy to prepare and can be customized with a variety of seasonings and flavorings to complement any main course. Here are some vegetable side dish ideas packed with nutrients:

1. **Roasted Vegetables**: Toss a mixture of seasonal vegetables such as carrots, broccoli, cauliflower, Brussels sprouts, and bell peppers with olive oil, garlic, and herbs such as thyme, rosemary, and oregano. Roast the vegetables in the oven until caramelized and tender for a flavorful and nutritious side dish that pairs well with grilled meats, roasted poultry, or fish.

2. **Sautéed Greens**: Heat olive oil in a skillet and sauté leafy greens such as spinach, kale, Swiss chard, or collard greens until wilted and tender. Season the greens with garlic, lemon juice, and red pepper flakes for added flavor and serve them as a nutritious accompaniment to pasta dishes, grilled chicken, or tofu.

3. **Steamed Asparagus with Lemon**: Steam fresh asparagus spears until crisp-tender, then drizzle them with olive oil and lemon juice and sprinkle them with sea salt and black pepper. Serve the steamed asparagus as a vibrant and refreshing side dish that pairs well with roasted salmon, grilled steak, or quinoa pilaf.

4. **Grilled Zucchini and Squash**: Slice zucchini and yellow squash into rounds and toss them with olive oil, balsamic vinegar, and Italian seasoning. Grill the zucchini and squash until charred and tender, then sprinkle them with grated Parmesan cheese and chopped fresh herbs such as basil or parsley for a flavorful and colorful side dish that's perfect for summer cookouts.

5. **Cauliflower Rice Pilaf**: Pulse cauliflower florets in a food processor until they resemble rice grains, then sauté the cauliflower rice with diced onions, carrots, celery, and garlic until tender. Season the cauliflower rice pilaf with curry powder, turmeric, and cumin for a fragrant and flavorful side dish that pairs well with grilled shrimp, chicken tikka masala, or tofu stir-fry.

6. **Stuffed Bell Peppers**: Cut bell peppers in half and remove the seeds and membranes, then stuff them with a mixture of cooked quinoa, black beans, corn, diced tomatoes, and chopped cilantro. Top the stuffed bell peppers with

shredded cheese and bake them until bubbly and golden brown for a hearty and nutritious side dish that's packed with protein and fiber.

7. **Balsamic Glazed Brussels Sprouts**: Roast halved Brussels sprouts in the oven until caramelized and tender, then drizzle them with a balsamic glaze made from balsamic vinegar, honey or maple syrup, and Dijon mustard. Toss the Brussels sprouts until evenly coated and serve them as a sweet and tangy side dish that pairs well with roasted pork tenderloin, grilled sausages, or lentil stew.

8. **Mushroom and Spinach Sauté**: Sauté sliced mushrooms and baby spinach in olive oil with minced garlic and shallots until the mushrooms are golden brown and the spinach is wilted. Season the mushroom and spinach sauté with salt, pepper, and a splash of balsamic vinegar for a flavorful and nutritious side dish that's perfect for serving alongside grilled steak, roasted chicken, or pasta.

By incorporating simple vegetable side dishes into your meals, you can increase your intake of nutrients and add vibrant colors and flavors to your plate. Experiment with different vegetables, seasonings, and cooking methods to create delicious and nutritious side dishes that complement any meal.

Whole Grain and Legume-Based Side Dishes for Balanced Nutrition

Whole grains and legumes are nutritious and versatile ingredients that can be used to create flavorful and satisfying side dishes that provide essential nutrients such as fiber, protein, vitamins, and minerals. Whole grain and legume-based side dishes are easy to prepare and can be customized with a variety of herbs, spices, and seasonings to complement any main course. Here are some ideas for whole grain and legume-based side dishes for balanced nutrition:

1. **Quinoa Salad**: Cook quinoa according to package instructions, then toss it with diced vegetables such as cucumbers, tomatoes, bell peppers, and red onions. Add chopped fresh herbs such as parsley, mint, and cilantro, and dress the quinoa salad with a lemon vinaigrette made from lemon juice, olive oil, garlic, and Dijon mustard for a refreshing and nutritious side dish that's perfect for picnics, barbecues, or potlucks.

2. **Brown Rice Pilaf**: Sauté diced onions, carrots, and celery in olive oil until softened, then add brown rice and cook until toasted. Gradually add vegetable broth and bring the mixture to a boil, then reduce the heat and simmer until the rice is tender and the liquid is absorbed. Stir in chopped almonds, dried cranberries, and chopped fresh parsley for a

flavorful and hearty side dish that pairs well with roasted chicken, grilled fish, or tofu.

3. **Lentil Salad**: Cook green or brown lentils until tender, then toss them with diced bell peppers, cherry tomatoes, cucumbers, and red onions. Add crumbled feta cheese, chopped fresh dill, and a squeeze of lemon juice, and season the lentil salad with salt, pepper, and a drizzle of olive oil for a protein-rich and satisfying side dish that's perfect for lunch or dinner.

4. **Chickpea Curry**: Sauté diced onions, garlic, and ginger in olive oil until softened, then add canned chickpeas, diced tomatoes, coconut milk, and curry powder. Simmer the mixture until heated through and the flavors have melded together, then stir in chopped spinach or kale for added nutrition and color. Serve the chickpea curry over cooked brown rice or quinoa for a flavorful and filling side dish that's perfect for vegetarians and meat-eaters alike.

5. **Black Bean and Corn Salad**: Combine canned black beans, cooked corn kernels, diced red bell peppers, chopped cilantro, and minced jalapeños in a bowl. Toss the mixture with lime juice, olive oil, cumin, and chili powder, and season with salt and pepper to taste. Serve the black bean and corn salad as a zesty and refreshing side dish that pairs well with grilled meats, fish tacos, or quesadillas.

6. **Barley Risotto**: Cook pearled barley in vegetable broth until tender, then stir in sautéed mushrooms, diced onions, minced garlic, and chopped fresh thyme. Finish the barley risotto with grated Parmesan cheese and a drizzle of balsamic glaze for a comforting and flavorful side dish that's perfect for serving alongside roasted vegetables, grilled steak, or baked chicken.

7. **Farro Salad**: Cook farro according to package instructions, then toss it with diced cucumbers, cherry tomatoes, Kalamata olives, and crumbled feta cheese. Add chopped fresh basil, oregano, and parsley, and dress the farro salad with a balsamic vinaigrette made from balsamic vinegar, olive oil, garlic, and Dijon mustard for a Mediterranean-inspired side dish that's bursting with flavor and nutrition.

8. **Split Pea Soup**: Simmer dried split peas with diced onions, carrots, celery, garlic, and vegetable broth until the peas are tender and the vegetables are soft. Puree the soup until smooth using an immersion blender or countertop blender, then season with salt, pepper, and a splash of lemon juice. Serve the split pea soup as a comforting and nourishing side dish that's perfect for chilly evenings or as a starter for a larger meal.

By incorporating whole grain and legume-based side dishes into your meals, you can increase your intake of fiber, protein, vitamins, and minerals while adding variety and flavor to your plate. Experiment with different grains, legumes, and flavorings to create delicious and nutritious side dishes that complement any meal.

Creative Ways to Add Flavor to Your Side Dish Repertoire

Adding flavor to side dishes can elevate a meal and make it more enjoyable and satisfying. By incorporating herbs, spices, condiments, and flavorful ingredients, you can transform simple side dishes into culinary delights that complement any main course. Here are some creative ways to add flavor to your side dish repertoire:

1. **Herb-Infused Olive Oil**: Make herb-infused olive oil by heating olive oil in a saucepan with fresh herbs such as rosemary, thyme, sage, or basil until fragrant. Remove the herbs and use the infused oil to drizzle over roasted vegetables, cooked grains, or grilled bread for a burst of flavor and aroma.

2. **Citrus Zest and Juice**: Add brightness and acidity to side dishes by incorporating citrus zest and juice. Grate the zest of lemons, limes, or oranges over cooked vegetables, salads, or grains, and squeeze fresh citrus juice over roasted meats, seafood, or tofu for a refreshing and tangy flavor boost.

3. **Toasted Nuts and Seeds**: Toast nuts and seeds such as almonds, walnuts, pumpkin seeds, or sesame seeds in a dry skillet until golden brown and fragrant. Sprinkle the toasted nuts and seeds over salads, grain dishes, or roasted vegetables for added crunch, flavor, and nutrition.

4. **Spice Blends and Seasonings**: Experiment with different spice blends and seasonings to add depth and complexity to side dishes. Mix together spices such as cumin, coriander, paprika, and chili powder to create a homemade taco seasoning for roasted sweet potatoes, black beans, and corn. Or use a blend of curry powder, turmeric, and ginger to season lentils, rice, and vegetables for a fragrant and flavorful Indian-inspired side dish.

5. **Fresh Herbs and Aromatics**: Finely chop fresh herbs such as parsley, cilantro, dill, or mint, and sprinkle them over cooked vegetables, grains, or salads for a burst of freshness and color. Sauté aromatics such as garlic, shallots, onions, or ginger in olive oil until softened and fragrant, then toss them with roasted vegetables, pasta, or couscous for added flavor and depth.

6. **Flavored Vinegars and Condiments**: Use flavored vinegars such as balsamic, apple cider, or red wine vinegar to dress salads, marinate vegetables, or drizzle over roasted meats. Experiment with condiments such as pesto, harissa, tahini, or

miso paste to add richness and complexity to side dishes such as roasted vegetables, grain salads, or stir-fries.

7. **Pickled and Fermented Foods**: Incorporate pickled and fermented foods such as pickles, sauerkraut, kimchi, or olives into side dishes to add acidity, tanginess, and probiotics. Serve pickled vegetables alongside grilled meats or fish, or toss fermented foods into grain salads or vegetable stir-fries for added flavor and gut health benefits.

8. **Umami-Rich Ingredients**: Enhance the savory flavor of side dishes by using umami-rich ingredients such as mushrooms, soy sauce, nutritional yeast, or Parmesan cheese. Sauté mushrooms until golden brown and caramelized, then toss them with cooked grains, pasta, or risotto for a hearty and satisfying side dish. Or sprinkle nutritional yeast or grated Parmesan cheese over roasted vegetables, salads, or soups for a savory and cheesy flavor boost.

By incorporating these creative ways to add flavor into your side dish repertoire, you can transform simple dishes into culinary masterpieces that complement any meal. Experiment with different ingredients, techniques, and flavor combinations to create side dishes that are delicious, satisfying, and memorable.

CHAPTER NINE

Dining Out and Socializing with Diabetes

Strategies for Making Healthy Choices When Eating Out

Eating out can be a challenge when you have diabetes, but with careful planning and smart choices, you can enjoy restaurant meals while managing your blood sugar levels effectively. Here are some strategies for making healthy choices when dining out:

1. **Research the Menu in Advance**: Many restaurants now provide their menus online, allowing you to review your options before you arrive. Look for dishes that are grilled, baked, or steamed rather than fried, and choose items that are rich in lean proteins, vegetables, and whole grains.

2. **Choose Lighter Options**: Opt for lighter fare such as salads, soups, and grilled or broiled seafood or poultry. Ask for dressings and sauces on the side so you can control the amount you use, and request steamed vegetables or a side salad instead of fries or chips.

3. **Control Portion Sizes**: Restaurant portions are often larger than what you would eat at home, so consider sharing an entrée with a dining companion or asking for a half portion. You can also ask for a to-go box when your meal arrives and set aside half of it to take home for later.

4. **Be Mindful of Carbohydrates**: Pay attention to carbohydrate-rich foods such as bread, pasta, rice, and potatoes, as they can cause spikes in blood sugar levels. Limit your intake of these foods or choose smaller portions, and opt for whole grain options when available.

5. **Watch Your Beverages**: Be cautious of sugary beverages such as soda, juice, and cocktails, as they can contain a significant amount of added sugars and carbohydrates. Stick to water, unsweetened tea or coffee, or diet beverages to help control your blood sugar levels.

6. **Ask Questions and Make Substitutions**: Don't be afraid to ask your server about the ingredients and preparation methods used in certain dishes, and request modifications to better suit your dietary needs. For example, you can ask for grilled chicken instead of fried, or steamed vegetables instead of mashed potatoes.

7. **Avoid Temptation**: Skip the breadbasket or chips and salsa that are often served before the meal, as they can add unnecessary calories and carbohydrates. Focus on enjoying the company of your dining companions rather than filling up on empty calories.

8. **Practice Portion Control with Desserts**: If you decide to indulge in dessert, consider sharing a sweet treat with your tablemates or opting for a lighter option such as fresh fruit

or sorbet. Alternatively, ask if the restaurant offers a sugar-free or low-carb dessert option.

By following these strategies for making healthy choices when dining out, you can enjoy restaurant meals while still managing your diabetes effectively. Remember to listen to your body and make choices that align with your dietary goals and preferences.

Tips for Navigating Social Events and Celebrations

Social events and celebrations often revolve around food, which can present challenges for individuals with diabetes. However, with some planning and preparation, you can navigate these occasions while still enjoying yourself. Here are some tips for navigating social events and celebrations with diabetes:

1. **Plan Ahead**: If you know you'll be attending a social event or celebration, plan your meals and snacks for the day accordingly to help manage your blood sugar levels. Consider eating a balanced meal or snack before you go to help prevent overeating or making unhealthy choices later on.

2. **Communicate with the Host**: If you're attending a gathering at someone's home, don't hesitate to communicate your dietary needs with the host in advance. Offer to bring a dish to share that aligns with your dietary preferences, or ask if

there will be options available that are suitable for your needs.

3. **Focus on Socializing**: Instead of making food the main focus of social events, focus on spending time with friends and loved ones. Engage in conversation, participate in activities, or offer to help with preparations or cleanup to keep yourself occupied and less tempted by food.

4. **Practice Portion Control**: Be mindful of portion sizes and resist the urge to overindulge, especially if there are tempting treats or high-calorie foods available. Choose smaller portions of your favorite foods and savor each bite, paying attention to hunger and fullness cues.

5. **Make Smart Choices**: Scan the buffet or food spread and identify healthier options such as fresh fruits, vegetables, lean proteins, and whole grains. Fill your plate with these nutrient-rich foods first before sampling higher-calorie or indulgent treats.

6. **Stay Hydrated**: Drink plenty of water throughout the event to stay hydrated and help prevent overeating. Avoid sugary beverages and alcohol, which can add unnecessary calories and affect blood sugar levels.

7. **Be Prepared for Peer Pressure**: Be prepared to politely decline offers of food or drinks that don't align with your

dietary goals, and don't be afraid to assertively communicate your needs if necessary. Remember that it's okay to prioritize your health and well-being.

8. **Bring Your Own Snacks**: If you're unsure about the food options available at a social event, consider bringing your own snacks or treats that you know are diabetes-friendly. This way, you'll have something to enjoy without feeling deprived or left out.

By following these tips for navigating social events and celebrations with diabetes, you can enjoy yourself while still managing your blood sugar levels effectively. Remember to focus on balance, moderation, and making choices that align with your health and wellness goals.

Communicating Your Dietary Needs Effectively

Communicating your dietary needs effectively is essential when dining out or attending social events, especially when you have specific dietary restrictions or health concerns such as diabetes. Here are some tips for effectively communicating your dietary needs:

1. **Be Clear and Specific**: Clearly communicate your dietary needs to restaurant staff or hosts by specifying any food allergies, intolerances, or health conditions such as diabetes. Provide specific instructions or requests if necessary, such as

asking for sauces or dressings on the side or requesting substitutions for certain ingredients.

2. **Ask Questions**: Don't hesitate to ask questions about menu items or food preparation methods to ensure they meet your dietary requirements. Inquire about ingredients, cooking techniques, and potential cross-contamination risks if you have concerns about allergens or other dietary restrictions.

3. **Use Positive Language**: Frame your dietary needs in a positive and constructive manner to avoid coming across as demanding or difficult. Use phrases such as "I need to avoid gluten due to a medical condition" or "Could you please help me find a low-carb option?" to convey your needs respectfully.

4. **Offer Suggestions**: If you're unsure about the available options, offer suggestions or alternatives that would better suit your dietary needs. For example, you can ask if a grilled chicken breast can be substituted for fried chicken, or if vegetables can be steamed instead of sautéed in butter.

5. **Express Appreciation**: Express gratitude to restaurant staff or hosts for accommodating your dietary needs and for their assistance in selecting suitable options. A simple thank you can go a long way in fostering positive communication and ensuring a pleasant dining experience for everyone involved.

6. **Provide Feedback**: If you encounter any issues or concerns with your meal, provide constructive feedback to restaurant staff or hosts in a polite and respectful manner. Offer suggestions for improvement or clarification to help them better understand your needs for future reference.

7. **Be Flexible**: While it's important to communicate your dietary needs effectively, it's also important to be flexible and open-minded when dining out or attending social events. Be willing to make compromises or adjustments if necessary, and focus on finding solutions that allow you to enjoy the experience without compromising your health.

8. **Educate Others**: Take the opportunity to educate others about your dietary needs and the reasons behind them, especially if they are unfamiliar with diabetes or other health conditions. By raising awareness and fostering understanding, you can help create a supportive and inclusive environment for everyone.

By effectively communicating your dietary needs, you can ensure that your meals are prepared in a way that supports your health and well-being while still enjoying dining out and socializing with others. Remember to be proactive, positive, and respectful in your interactions, and advocate for yourself to receive the accommodations you need.

CHAPTER TEN

Meal Planning and Preparation for Success

Practical Tips for Meal Planning and Grocery Shopping

Meal planning and grocery shopping are essential components of maintaining a healthy diet, especially for individuals with diabetes. By planning ahead and making thoughtful choices at the grocery store, you can set yourself up for success in managing your blood sugar levels and achieving your dietary goals. Here are some practical tips for meal planning and grocery shopping:

1. **Set Aside Time for Planning**: Dedicate a specific time each week to plan your meals and create a grocery list. Consider factors such as your schedule, dietary preferences, and nutritional needs when deciding what to eat for the week ahead.

2. **Start with a Template**: Use a meal planning template or calendar to map out your meals for each day of the week, including breakfast, lunch, dinner, and snacks. Consider incorporating a variety of foods from different food groups to ensure balanced nutrition.

3. **Plan for Leftovers**: Embrace leftovers as a time-saving strategy by intentionally cooking extra portions of meals that can be enjoyed as leftovers for lunch or dinner later in the

week. This can help reduce food waste and simplify meal preparation on busy days.

4. **Focus on Nutrient-Rich Foods**: Build your meals around nutrient-rich foods such as fruits, vegetables, whole grains, lean proteins, and healthy fats. Aim to fill your grocery cart with a colorful assortment of fresh produce, whole grains, and lean proteins to support your overall health and well-being.

5. **Read Labels Carefully**: When grocery shopping, read food labels carefully to check for added sugars, sodium, and unhealthy fats. Choose products with minimal added sugars and opt for lower sodium options whenever possible to support heart health and blood sugar control.

6. **Shop the Perimeter of the Store**: In general, the perimeter of the grocery store is where you'll find fresh produce, lean proteins, dairy products, and whole grains. Focus your shopping efforts on these areas to prioritize nutrient-dense foods and minimize exposure to processed and packaged foods.

7. **Stock Up on Staples**: Keep your pantry, refrigerator, and freezer stocked with staple ingredients that can be used to create a variety of meals and snacks. Examples include canned beans, whole grains, frozen vegetables, nuts and seeds, herbs and spices, and healthy cooking oils.

8. **Plan for Special Occasions and Cravings**: Allow yourself flexibility in your meal planning to accommodate special occasions, cravings, or spontaneous dining opportunities. Incorporate occasional treats or indulgences in moderation while staying mindful of portion sizes and overall dietary balance.

9. **Use Technology to Your Advantage**: Take advantage of meal planning apps, online recipe databases, and grocery delivery services to streamline the meal planning and grocery shopping process. These tools can help save time and energy while ensuring that you have access to nutritious foods that align with your dietary goals.

10. **Stay Organized**: Keep your meal plan, grocery list, and recipes organized in a centralized location such as a notebook, smartphone app, or online document. Refer to your meal plan and grocery list throughout the week to stay on track and avoid last-minute decisions or impulse purchases.

By incorporating these practical tips into your meal planning and grocery shopping routine, you can make healthier choices, save time and money, and set yourself up for success in managing your diabetes and overall well-being.

Batch Cooking and Freezing Meals for Convenience

Batch cooking and freezing meals are excellent strategies for saving time and ensuring that you always have nutritious meals on hand, especially on busy days when cooking from scratch may not be feasible. By preparing large batches of food ahead of time and portioning them out for future use, you can streamline meal preparation and reduce the temptation to rely on convenience foods or takeout. Here are some tips for batch cooking and freezing meals for convenience:

1. **Choose Recipes Wisely**: Select recipes that lend themselves well to batch cooking and freezing, such as soups, stews, casseroles, and chili. These types of dishes often improve in flavor over time and can be easily portioned out and reheated as needed.

2. **Invest in Storage Containers**: Purchase a variety of high-quality storage containers in different sizes to accommodate batch-cooked meals and individual portions. Opt for containers that are freezer-safe, microwave-safe, and stackable for easy storage and organization.

3. **Label and Date Everything**: Label each container with the name of the dish and the date it was prepared to help you keep track of what's in your freezer and how long it has been

stored. Use a permanent marker or removable labels that won't smudge or fade over time.

4. **Cool Foods Properly**: Allow batch-cooked foods to cool completely before transferring them to the refrigerator or freezer to prevent bacterial growth and maintain food safety. Divide large batches into smaller portions to speed up the cooling process and reduce the risk of spoilage.

5. **Use Freezer-Friendly Ingredients**: Choose ingredients that freeze well and maintain their texture and flavor after thawing, such as cooked grains, beans, lentils, vegetables, and lean proteins. Avoid ingredients that may become mushy or lose their quality when frozen, such as raw tomatoes, lettuce, or dairy-based sauces.

6. **Consider Meal Components**: Batch cook individual components of meals, such as cooked grains, roasted vegetables, grilled chicken, and homemade sauces or dressings, and assemble them into complete meals when ready to eat. This allows for greater flexibility and customization based on your preferences and dietary needs.

7. **Rotate Your Stock**: Practice first in, first out (FIFO) inventory management to ensure that older items are used up before newer ones. Periodically review your freezer inventory and plan meals around ingredients that need to be used up to minimize food waste.

8. **Thaw Safely**: Thaw frozen meals safely in the refrigerator overnight or use the defrost setting on your microwave for quicker thawing. Avoid thawing foods at room temperature, as this can increase the risk of bacterial growth and foodborne illness.

9. **Reheat Properly**: Reheat frozen meals thoroughly to an internal temperature of 165°F (74°C) to ensure food safety. Use a microwave, stovetop, or oven to reheat meals evenly, stirring or rotating as needed to prevent hot spots and ensure even heating.

10. **Get Creative with Leftovers**: Use batch-cooked meals and frozen leftovers as building blocks for new dishes and recipes. Incorporate leftover chili into tacos or baked potatoes, add cooked grains to salads or stir-fries, or repurpose roasted vegetables into soups or omelets for added variety and flavor.

By incorporating batch cooking and freezing meals into your meal planning routine, you can save time, reduce stress, and ensure that you always have nutritious meals available to enjoy, even on your busiest days.

Strategies for Portion Control and Balanced Eating

Portion control is an important aspect of managing diabetes and maintaining a healthy weight. By controlling portion sizes and practicing balanced eating habits, you can better regulate your blood sugar levels, improve insulin sensitivity, and support overall health and well-being. Here are some strategies for portion control and balanced eating:

1. **Use Portion-Controlled Plates and Utensils**: Invest in portion-controlled plates, bowls, and utensils that are designed to help you visualize appropriate serving sizes for different food groups. These tools can make portion control easier and more intuitive, especially for individuals who struggle with estimating portion sizes.

2. **Practice the Plate Method**: Use the plate method as a simple and effective way to balance your meals and control portion sizes. Fill half of your plate with non-starchy vegetables such as leafy greens, broccoli, or bell peppers, one-quarter with lean protein such as chicken, fish, or tofu, and one-quarter with whole grains or starchy vegetables such as brown rice, quinoa, or sweet potatoes.

3. **Measure Portions Accurately**: Use measuring cups, spoons, or a kitchen scale to measure portion sizes of foods that are easy to overeat, such as grains, nuts, seeds, and snacks. Be

mindful of serving sizes listed on food labels and adjust your portions accordingly to avoid unintentional overconsumption of calories and carbohydrates.

4. **Listen to Your Hunger and Fullness Cues**: Pay attention to your body's hunger and fullness cues to help you determine when to eat and when to stop. Eat slowly and mindfully, savoring each bite and stopping when you feel satisfied rather than overly full. Avoid distractions such as television or electronic devices while eating to focus on your meal and prevent mindless overeating.

5. **Eat Balanced Meals and Snacks**: Aim for balanced meals and snacks that contain a combination of carbohydrates, protein, and healthy fats to help stabilize blood sugar levels and promote satiety. Include a variety of nutrient-rich foods from different food groups to ensure that your meals are both satisfying and nourishing.

6. **Practice Mindful Eating**: Practice mindful eating by paying attention to the taste, texture, and aroma of your food, as well as the sensations of hunger and fullness in your body. Avoid eating on autopilot or in response to external cues such as stress, boredom, or social pressure, and instead focus on eating with intention and awareness.

7. **Control Portions of High-Calorie Foods**: Limit portions of high-calorie or high-fat foods such as fried foods, sweets,

desserts, and processed snacks, which can contribute to weight gain and negatively impact blood sugar control. Enjoy these foods occasionally and in moderation, and be mindful of portion sizes to avoid excess calories and carbohydrates.

8. **Plan Ahead for Eating Out**: When dining out or ordering takeout, plan ahead by reviewing the menu and choosing healthier options that align with your dietary goals. Consider splitting an entrée with a dining companion, ordering a smaller portion size, or requesting substitutions or modifications to make the meal more diabetes-friendly.

9. **Be Flexible and Forgiving**: Remember that no one is perfect, and occasional deviations from your meal plan or portion control goals are normal and to be expected. Be kind to yourself and practice self-compassion if you overindulge or make choices that aren't in line with your health goals. Focus on making positive changes over time and celebrate your progress along the way.

10. **Seek Support and Accountability**: Enlist the support of friends, family members, or a registered dietitian to help you stay accountable to your portion control and balanced eating goals. Share your successes and challenges with others, and celebrate small victories along your journey to better health.

By incorporating these strategies for portion control and balanced eating into your daily routine, you can better manage your diabetes, improve your overall health, and achieve your dietary goals. Remember to be patient with yourself and take small, sustainable steps toward building healthy eating habits that last a lifetime.

CHAPTER 11

DDIET FOR DIABETES

Mediterranean Diet:

Definition:

The Mediterranean diet is inspired by the traditional dietary patterns of countries bordering the Mediterranean Sea. It emphasizes whole, minimally processed foods such as fruits, vegetables, whole grains, nuts, seeds, legumes, fish, and olive oil. It limits red meat and sweets, while encouraging moderate consumption of dairy products, poultry, and eggs.

Ingredients:

- Fruits: Berries, apples, oranges, grapes, etc.

- Vegetables: Spinach, tomatoes, peppers, onions, etc.

- Whole Grains: Whole wheat bread, brown rice, quinoa, oats, etc.

- Nuts and Seeds: Almonds, walnuts, flaxseeds, chia seeds, etc.

- Legumes: Chickpeas, lentils, beans, etc.

- Fish and Seafood: Salmon, tuna, shrimp, etc.

- Olive Oil: Extra virgin olive oil for cooking and dressing.

- Herbs and Spices: Basil, oregano, garlic, cumin, etc.

Instructions/How to Prepare:

1. Base meals around plant-based foods like fruits, vegetables, whole grains, and legumes.

2. Use olive oil as the primary source of fat for cooking and dressing salads.

3. Incorporate fish and seafood into your diet regularly, aiming for at least two servings per week.

4. Enjoy moderate amounts of poultry, eggs, and dairy products, such as yogurt and cheese.

5. Limit red meat consumption to a few times per month.

6. Snack on nuts and seeds for a healthy source of fats and protein.

7. Flavor meals with herbs and spices instead of salt.

8. Drink plenty of water and enjoy a moderate amount of red wine if desired (optional).

DASH Diet (Dietary Approaches to Stop Hypertension):

Definition:

The DASH diet is specifically designed to help lower blood pressure and reduce the risk of hypertension. It emphasizes fruits, vegetables, whole grains, and lean proteins while limiting sodium, saturated fats, and sweets.

Ingredients:

- Fruits: Berries, bananas, apples, oranges, etc.

- Vegetables: Leafy greens, carrots, broccoli, bell peppers, etc.

- Whole Grains: Brown rice, whole wheat bread, quinoa, oats, barley, etc.

- Lean Proteins: Chicken breast, turkey, fish, tofu, beans, lentils, etc.

- Dairy: Low-fat or fat-free milk, yogurt, cheese, etc.

- Nuts and Seeds: Almonds, pistachios, sunflower seeds, etc.

- Healthy Fats: Olive oil, avocado, nuts, seeds, etc.

Instructions/How to Prepare:

1. Focus on incorporating plenty of fruits and vegetables into your meals and snacks.

2. Choose whole grains over refined grains whenever possible.

3. Opt for lean proteins such as poultry, fish, tofu, and legumes.

4. Limit high-fat dairy products and opt for low-fat or fat-free options.

5. Include nuts and seeds as snacks or in salads for added nutrients and healthy fats.

6. Use herbs, spices, and citrus juices to flavor foods instead of salt.

7. Avoid processed and high-sodium foods like canned soups, packaged snacks, and fast food.

8. Cook meals at home whenever possible to have better control over ingredients and portion sizes.

9. Aim to limit sweets and sugary beverages, opting for natural sweeteners like fruit when craving something sweet.

10.   Stay hydrated by drinking plenty of water throughout the day.

Low-Carb Diet:

Definition:

A low-carb diet involves reducing carbohydrate intake while increasing the consumption of protein and healthy fats. This diet aims to control insulin levels, promote weight loss, and improve overall health by limiting foods high in carbohydrates such as bread, pasta, rice, and sugary snacks.

Ingredients:

- Protein Sources: Meat, poultry, fish, tofu, tempeh, eggs.

- Non-Starchy Vegetables: Leafy greens, broccoli, cauliflower, zucchini, bell peppers.

- Healthy Fats: Avocado, nuts, seeds, olive oil, coconut oil.

- Dairy: Cheese, Greek yogurt, cottage cheese (in moderation).

- Low-Carb Fruits: Berries, avocados, tomatoes, lemons, limes.

- Herbs and Spices: Basil, oregano, garlic, turmeric, cumin.

- Sweeteners (optional): Stevia, erythritol, monk fruit.

Instructions/How to Prepare:

1. Focus on whole, unprocessed foods.

2. Limit carbohydrate intake to around 20-50 grams per day, depending on individual needs and goals.

3. Include protein-rich foods in each meal to promote satiety and muscle maintenance.

4. Fill up on non-starchy vegetables to increase fiber intake and provide essential vitamins and minerals.

5. Incorporate healthy fats into your diet for energy and to keep you feeling full.

6. Be mindful of hidden carbs in sauces, condiments, and processed foods.

7. Drink plenty of water to stay hydrated and support overall health.

8. Experiment with low-carb recipes and meal prep to make adhering to the diet easier and more enjoyable.

Ketogenic Diet (Keto Diet):

Definition:

The ketogenic diet is a very low-carb, high-fat diet that forces the body to enter a state of ketosis, where it primarily burns fat for fuel instead of carbohydrates. This diet has been used for decades to treat epilepsy and has gained popularity for weight loss and improving metabolic health.

Ingredients:

- Healthy Fats: Avocado, coconut oil, olive oil, butter, ghee, fatty fish.

- Protein Sources: Meat, poultry, fish, eggs, tofu, tempeh.

- Non-Starchy Vegetables: Leafy greens, broccoli, cauliflower, zucchini, asparagus.

- Full-Fat Dairy: Cheese, heavy cream, Greek yogurt (in moderation).

- Nuts and Seeds: Macadamia nuts, almonds, chia seeds, flaxseeds.

- Low-Carb Fruits: Berries (in moderation), avocado.

- Herbs and Spices: Turmeric, ginger, cinnamon, garlic, thyme.

- Sweeteners (in moderation): Stevia, erythritol, monk fruit.

Instructions/How to Prepare:

1. Keep carbohydrate intake extremely low, typically below 20-50 grams per day to induce and maintain ketosis.

2. Consume moderate amounts of protein, as excessive protein intake can potentially hinder ketosis.

3. Base meals around healthy fats, such as avocados, olive oil, and fatty fish.

4. Incorporate non-starchy vegetables to provide essential nutrients and fiber while keeping carbohydrate intake low.

5. Be mindful of hidden carbs in foods and beverages, including sauces, dressings, and flavored beverages.

6. Stay hydrated by drinking plenty of water, as dehydration can occur more easily on a ketogenic diet.

7. Monitor ketone levels using urine strips, blood tests, or breath meters if desired, to ensure you are in ketosis.

8. Experiment with keto-friendly recipes and meal planning to maintain variety and enjoyment while following the diet.

Plant-Based Diet:

Definition:

A plant-based diet primarily consists of foods derived from plants, such as fruits, vegetables, grains, nuts, seeds, and legumes. It emphasizes whole, minimally processed foods while minimizing or eliminating animal products. The focus is on incorporating a variety of plant foods to promote health and well-being.

Ingredients:

- Fruits: Berries, apples, oranges, bananas, etc.

- Vegetables: Leafy greens, broccoli, carrots, bell peppers, etc.

- Whole Grains: Brown rice, quinoa, oats, barley, whole wheat bread, etc.

- Legumes: Chickpeas, lentils, black beans, kidney beans, etc.

- Nuts and Seeds: Almonds, walnuts, chia seeds, flaxseeds, pumpkin seeds, etc.

- Plant-Based Proteins: Tofu, tempeh, seitan, edamame, plant-based protein powders, etc.

- Healthy Fats: Avocado, olive oil, coconut oil, nuts, seeds, etc.

Instructions/How to Prepare:

1. Base meals around a variety of whole plant foods, including fruits, vegetables, whole grains, legumes, nuts, and seeds.

2. Incorporate a rainbow of colorful fruits and vegetables to ensure a diverse array of nutrients.

3. Include plant-based proteins such as tofu, tempeh, and legumes in meals to meet protein needs.

4. Choose whole grains over refined grains for added fiber and nutrients.

5. Experiment with different cooking methods, such as steaming, roasting, sautéing, and grilling, to enhance flavor and texture.

6. Use herbs, spices, and condiments to add flavor to dishes without relying on animal products.

7. Be mindful of nutrient needs, particularly vitamin B12, vitamin D, omega-3 fatty acids, iron, calcium, and zinc, and consider supplementation if necessary.

8. Stay hydrated by drinking plenty of water throughout the day.

9. Plan balanced meals and snacks to ensure adequate intake of essential nutrients.

10. Enjoy plant-based alternatives to dairy and meat products, such as plant-based milk, cheese, yogurt, and meat substitutes, if desired.

Vegan Diet:

Definition:

A vegan diet excludes all animal products, including meat, poultry, fish, dairy, eggs, and honey. It is based entirely on plant foods and emphasizes cruelty-free living and environmental sustainability.

Ingredients:

- Fruits: Berries, apples, oranges, mangoes, etc.
- Vegetables: Spinach, kale, tomatoes, onions, mushrooms, etc.
- Whole Grains: Quinoa, brown rice, barley, whole wheat pasta, etc.
- Legumes: Chickpeas, black beans, lentils, kidney beans, etc.
- Nuts and Seeds: Almonds, cashews, sunflower seeds, chia seeds, etc.
- Plant-Based Proteins: Tofu, tempeh, seitan, soy-based meat substitutes, etc.
- Healthy Fats: Avocado, olive oil, coconut oil, nuts, seeds, etc.
- Plant-Based Dairy Alternatives: Almond milk, coconut milk, soy milk, vegan cheese, vegan yogurt, etc.

Instructions/How to Prepare:

1. Build meals around plant foods, including fruits, vegetables, whole grains, legumes, nuts, and seeds.

2. Ensure adequate protein intake by including sources such as tofu, tempeh, legumes, and plant-based meat substitutes.

3. Use plant-based milk, cheese, and yogurt alternatives in place of dairy products.

4. Experiment with vegan cooking techniques and recipes to discover new flavors and textures.

5. Pay attention to nutrient needs, especially vitamin B12, vitamin D, omega-3 fatty acids, iron, calcium, and zinc, and consider supplementation if necessary.

6. Read labels carefully to avoid hidden animal ingredients in processed foods and beverages.

7. Be mindful of cross-contamination when preparing and consuming food to prevent unintentional consumption of animal products.

8. Explore vegan-friendly restaurants and eateries or plan ahead when dining out to ensure vegan options are available.

9. Connect with vegan communities and resources for support, recipe ideas, and lifestyle tips.

10. Embrace the ethical and environmental principles of veganism beyond diet by choosing cruelty-free and

sustainable products in other areas of life, such as clothing, cosmetics, and household items.

Vegetarian Diet:

Definition:

A vegetarian diet excludes meat, poultry, and seafood, but includes plant-based foods such as fruits, vegetables, grains, nuts, seeds, and dairy products. There are different variations of vegetarianism, including lacto-vegetarian (includes dairy but not eggs), ovo-vegetarian (includes eggs but not dairy), and lacto-ovo-vegetarian (includes both dairy and eggs).

Ingredients:

- Fruits: Berries, apples, oranges, bananas, etc.
- Vegetables: Leafy greens, broccoli, carrots, bell peppers, etc.
- Whole Grains: Brown rice, quinoa, oats, barley, whole wheat bread, etc.
- Legumes: Chickpeas, lentils, black beans, kidney beans, etc.
- Nuts and Seeds: Almonds, walnuts, chia seeds, flaxseeds, pumpkin seeds, etc.
- Dairy: Milk, yogurt, cheese, butter, etc. (depending on the type of vegetarianism)

- Plant-Based Proteins: Tofu, tempeh, seitan, edamame, etc.

- Healthy Fats: Avocado, olive oil, coconut oil, nuts, seeds, etc.

Instructions/How to Prepare:

1. Base meals around a variety of plant foods, including fruits, vegetables, whole grains, legumes, nuts, and seeds.

2. Incorporate plant-based proteins such as tofu, tempeh, legumes, nuts, and seeds into meals to meet protein needs.

3. Choose whole grains over refined grains for added fiber and nutrients.

4. Experiment with different cooking methods, such as steaming, roasting, sautéing, and grilling, to enhance flavor and texture.

5. Use herbs, spices, and condiments to add flavor to dishes without relying on meat.

6. Be mindful of nutrient needs, especially vitamin B12, vitamin D, omega-3 fatty acids, iron, calcium, and zinc, and consider supplementation if necessary.

7. Stay hydrated by drinking plenty of water throughout the day.

8. Plan balanced meals and snacks to ensure adequate intake of essential nutrients.

9. Explore vegetarian cooking techniques and recipes to discover new flavors and textures.

10.   Connect with vegetarian communities and resources for support, recipe ideas, and lifestyle tips.

Atkins Diet:

Definition:

The Atkins diet is a low-carbohydrate, high-fat diet designed for weight loss and improving overall health. It involves reducing carbohydrate intake while increasing the consumption of protein and healthy fats. The diet is divided into four phases: induction, balancing, fine-tuning, and maintenance.

Ingredients:

- Protein Sources: Meat, poultry, fish, eggs, tofu, tempeh, etc.

- Non-Starchy Vegetables: Leafy greens, broccoli, cauliflower, zucchini, bell peppers, etc.

- Healthy Fats: Avocado, olive oil, coconut oil, butter, ghee, fatty fish, etc.

- Full-Fat Dairy (in moderation): Cheese, Greek yogurt, heavy cream, etc.

- Nuts and Seeds (in moderation): Almonds, walnuts, chia seeds, flaxseeds, etc.

- Low-Carb Fruits (in moderation): Berries, avocados, tomatoes, etc.

- Herbs and Spices: Basil, oregano, garlic, turmeric, cumin, etc.

Instructions/How to Prepare:

1. Start with the induction phase, which restricts carbohydrate intake to 20-25 grams per day for two weeks to induce ketosis.

2. Base meals around protein-rich foods such as meat, poultry, fish, eggs, and tofu.

3. Include non-starchy vegetables to provide essential nutrients and fiber while keeping carbohydrate intake low.

4. Incorporate healthy fats into your diet for energy and to keep you feeling full.

5. Gradually increase carbohydrate intake during the balancing, fine-tuning, and maintenance phases while monitoring weight and overall health.

6. Be mindful of portion sizes and track carbohydrate intake to stay within the recommended limits for each phase.

7. Stay hydrated by drinking plenty of water throughout the day.

8. Experiment with low-carb recipes and meal planning to maintain variety and enjoyment while following the diet.

9. Consider working with a healthcare professional or registered dietitian to personalize the diet plan and ensure nutritional adequacy.

10. Monitor progress and make adjustments as needed to achieve weight loss and health goals.

South Beach Diet:

Definition:

The South Beach Diet is a popular weight-loss program that emphasizes the consumption of lean protein, healthy fats, and low-glycemic carbohydrates. It's divided into three phases: Phase 1, which eliminates most carbs to jump-start weight loss; Phase 2, which reintroduces some carbs while continuing weight loss; and Phase 3, which focuses on maintaining weight loss with a balanced diet.

Ingredients:

- Lean Proteins: Chicken breast, turkey, fish, seafood, lean cuts of beef and pork.

- Healthy Fats: Olive oil, avocado, nuts, seeds, fatty fish like salmon and mackerel.

- Low-Glycemic Carbohydrates: Non-starchy vegetables (e.g., spinach, broccoli, cauliflower), whole grains (e.g., quinoa, barley), legumes (e.g., beans, lentils).

- Low-Fat Dairy: Greek yogurt, skim milk, low-fat cheese.

Instructions/How to Prepare:

1. Phase 1: Eliminate most carbohydrates, including fruits, grains, and starchy vegetables. Focus on lean proteins, non-starchy vegetables, and healthy fats. Drink plenty of water and avoid processed foods and added sugars.

2. Phase 2: Gradually reintroduce some carbohydrates, such as fruits and whole grains, while continuing to prioritize lean proteins and healthy fats. Monitor portion sizes and continue to avoid refined sugars and processed foods.

3. Phase 3: Transition to a balanced diet that includes a variety of foods from all food groups. Focus on portion control, mindful eating, and regular physical activity to maintain weight loss and overall health.

Paleo Diet:

Definition:

The Paleo diet, also known as the Paleolithic or caveman diet, is based on the presumed diet of ancient humans during the Paleolithic era. It emphasizes whole foods that would have been available to our hunter-gatherer ancestors, such as lean meats, fish, fruits, vegetables, nuts, and seeds, while excluding processed foods, grains, legumes, and dairy products.

Ingredients:

- Lean Meats: Beef, chicken, turkey, pork, lamb, etc.

- Fish and Seafood: Salmon, trout, shrimp, shellfish, etc.

- Fruits: Berries, apples, oranges, bananas, etc.

- Vegetables: Leafy greens, broccoli, carrots, peppers, onions, etc.

- Nuts and Seeds: Almonds, walnuts, cashews, sunflower seeds, etc.

- Healthy Fats: Avocado, olive oil, coconut oil, ghee.

- Herbs and Spices: Basil, oregano, garlic, turmeric, cinnamon, etc.

Instructions/How to Prepare:

1. Base meals around lean proteins, including meat, fish, and seafood.

2. Incorporate a variety of colorful fruits and vegetables for essential vitamins, minerals, and fiber.

3. Include nuts and seeds as snacks or to add texture and flavor to meals.

4. Use healthy fats like olive oil, avocado, and coconut oil for cooking and dressing.

5. Avoid processed foods, grains, legumes, dairy products, refined sugars, and artificial additives.

6. Experiment with cooking methods such as grilling, baking, and sautéing to enhance flavor and texture.

7. Stay hydrated by drinking plenty of water throughout the day.

8. Listen to your body's hunger and fullness cues and eat mindfully.

9. Be aware of portion sizes and adjust based on individual energy needs and activity levels.

10. Focus on whole, nutrient-dense foods and prioritize quality over quantity.

Whole30 Diet:

Definition:

The Whole30 diet is a 30-day elimination diet designed to reset your body and identify potential food sensitivities. It involves removing certain food groups known to cause inflammation and digestive issues, such as sugar, grains, dairy, legumes, and processed foods, for 30 days. After the elimination period, foods are gradually reintroduced to identify which ones may be causing adverse reactions.

Ingredients:

- Protein Sources: Meat, poultry, fish, seafood, eggs.

- Vegetables: Leafy greens, cruciferous vegetables, peppers, squash, etc.

- Fruits: Berries, apples, oranges, bananas, etc.

- Healthy Fats: Avocado, olive oil, coconut oil, nuts, seeds.

- Herbs and Spices: Basil, oregano, garlic, turmeric, cinnamon, etc.

Instructions/How to Prepare:

1. Eliminate sugar, grains, dairy, legumes, and processed foods from your diet for 30 days.

2. Base meals around protein sources, including meat, poultry, fish, seafood, and eggs.

3. Include a variety of vegetables for essential vitamins, minerals, and fiber.

4. Incorporate fruits as snacks or to add natural sweetness to meals.

5. Use healthy fats like avocado, olive oil, and coconut oil for cooking and dressing.

6. Experiment with herbs and spices to enhance flavor without added sugars or artificial additives.

7. Be mindful of hidden sources of sugar and processed ingredients in condiments and packaged foods.

8. Read labels carefully and opt for whole, minimally processed foods.

9. Stay hydrated by drinking plenty of water throughout the day.

10. After the 30-day elimination period, reintroduce eliminated foods one at a time and monitor for any adverse reactions or changes in symptoms.

Low-Glycemic Index Diet:

Definition:

The Low-Glycemic Index (GI) diet focuses on consuming foods that have a low glycemic index, which means they cause a slower and more gradual increase in blood sugar levels. This diet can help stabilize blood sugar, improve insulin sensitivity, and promote weight loss. Foods with a low GI typically include non-starchy vegetables, whole grains, lean proteins, and healthy fats.

Ingredients:

- Non-Starchy Vegetables: Leafy greens, broccoli, cauliflower, peppers, carrots, etc.

- Whole Grains: Quinoa, barley, bulgur, oats, brown rice, etc.

- Lean Proteins: Chicken breast, turkey, fish, tofu, tempeh, beans, lentils.

- Healthy Fats: Avocado, olive oil, nuts, seeds, fatty fish like salmon.

- Low-Glycemic Fruits (in moderation): Berries, apples, oranges, pears, etc.

- Herbs and Spices: Basil, oregano, garlic, turmeric, cinnamon, etc.

Instructions/How to Prepare:

1. Choose whole, minimally processed foods with a low glycemic index.

2. Base meals around non-starchy vegetables, whole grains, and lean proteins.

3. Incorporate healthy fats like avocado, olive oil, nuts, and seeds for satiety and flavor.

4. Limit high-glycemic foods such as refined grains, sugary snacks, and sweetened beverages.

5. Include low-glycemic fruits in moderation, focusing on berries, apples, and citrus fruits.

6. Be mindful of portion sizes and avoid overeating, even with low-GI foods.

7. Experiment with cooking methods such as steaming, roasting, and sautéing to enhance flavor and texture.

8. Eat balanced meals that combine protein, carbohydrates, and healthy fats to promote satiety and stabilize blood sugar levels.

9. Monitor blood sugar levels if necessary and adjust your diet accordingly.

10.   Stay hydrated by drinking plenty of water throughout the day.

Low-Fat Diet:

Definition:

A low-fat diet is characterized by reducing the intake of dietary fats, particularly saturated fats and trans fats, to promote heart health, manage weight, and reduce the risk of certain chronic diseases such as cardiovascular disease. This diet typically involves limiting foods high in fat and choosing lean protein sources, whole grains, fruits, vegetables, and low-fat dairy products.

Ingredients:

- Lean Proteins: Skinless poultry, lean cuts of beef and pork, fish, tofu, tempeh, legumes.

- Whole Grains: Brown rice, quinoa, barley, whole wheat bread, oats, whole grain pasta.

- Fruits: Berries, apples, oranges, bananas, grapes, etc.

- Vegetables: Leafy greens, broccoli, carrots, bell peppers, tomatoes, etc.

- Low-Fat or Fat-Free Dairy: Skim milk, low-fat yogurt, reduced-fat cheese.

- Healthy Fats (in moderation): Avocado, nuts, seeds, olive oil.

Instructions/How to Prepare:

1. Choose lean protein sources such as poultry, fish, tofu, and legumes instead of high-fat meats.

2. Opt for whole grains like brown rice, quinoa, and whole wheat bread over refined grains.

3. Include a variety of fruits and vegetables in your meals and snacks for added vitamins, minerals, and fiber.

4. Select low-fat or fat-free dairy products to reduce saturated fat intake.

5. Limit added fats and oils, and use healthier cooking methods such as baking, grilling, steaming, or boiling.

6. Be mindful of portion sizes to avoid overconsumption of calories, even with low-fat foods.

7. Read food labels to identify hidden sources of fat and choose lower-fat options when available.

8. Incorporate healthy fats like avocado, nuts, and olive oil in moderation for flavor and satiety.

9. Stay hydrated by drinking plenty of water throughout the day.

10.   Focus on overall dietary patterns rather than just reducing fat intake, and aim for a balanced diet that includes a variety of nutrient-dense foods.

High-Fiber Diet:

Definition:

A high-fiber diet focuses on increasing the intake of dietary fiber, which offers numerous health benefits such as improving digestion, promoting satiety, stabilizing blood sugar levels, and reducing the risk of chronic diseases such as heart disease, diabetes, and certain cancers. This diet emphasizes whole, unprocessed foods rich in fiber, including fruits, vegetables, whole grains, legumes, nuts, and seeds.

Ingredients:

- Whole Grains: Oats, barley, quinoa, brown rice, whole wheat bread, whole grain pasta.

- Fruits: Berries, apples, oranges, pears, bananas, avocados, etc.

- Vegetables: Leafy greens, broccoli, carrots, Brussels sprouts, sweet potatoes, etc.

- Legumes: Lentils, chickpeas, black beans, kidney beans, peas, etc.

- Nuts and Seeds: Almonds, chia seeds, flaxseeds, pumpkin seeds, sunflower seeds, etc.

- Healthy Fats: Avocado, nuts, seeds, olive oil, flaxseed oil.

Instructions/How to Prepare:

1. Incorporate a variety of whole grains, fruits, vegetables, legumes, nuts, and seeds into your meals and snacks.

2. Choose whole fruits and vegetables over fruit juices and refined grains to maximize fiber intake.

3. Include high-fiber foods such as beans, lentils, and chickpeas in soups, salads, and main dishes.

4. Replace refined grains with whole grains in recipes and meals, such as swapping white rice for brown rice or white bread for whole wheat bread.

5. Snack on raw vegetables with hummus or nut butter for a fiber-rich snack.

6. Add nuts, seeds, and avocado to salads, yogurt, or smoothies for added fiber and healthy fats.

7. Be sure to drink plenty of water throughout the day to help move fiber through the digestive tract and prevent constipation.

8. Gradually increase fiber intake to allow your digestive system to adjust and minimize discomfort.

9. Monitor portion sizes, especially with high-calorie fiber-rich foods like nuts and seeds.

10. Aim to include a variety of fiber sources in your diet to ensure you're getting a balance of soluble and insoluble fiber, which offer different health benefits.

Flexitarian Diet:

Definition:

The Flexitarian diet is a flexible approach to eating that emphasizes plant-based foods while allowing for occasional consumption of meat and other animal products. It encourages individuals to primarily eat fruits, vegetables, whole grains, legumes, nuts, and seeds, while minimizing intake of processed foods, sugar, and refined grains. The diet is flexible and adaptable, making it suitable for various lifestyles and preferences.

Ingredients:

- Plant-Based Foods: Fruits, vegetables, whole grains, legumes, nuts, seeds.

- Lean Proteins: Tofu, tempeh, beans, lentils, chickpeas, edamame.

- Healthy Fats: Avocado, nuts, seeds, olive oil.

- Dairy and Eggs (optional): Greek yogurt, eggs, low-fat cheese.

- Occasional Meat and Fish: Lean cuts of poultry, fish, seafood (optional).

Instructions/How to Prepare:

1. Base meals around plant-based foods such as fruits, vegetables, whole grains, legumes, nuts, and seeds.

2. Include a variety of colorful fruits and vegetables to ensure a diverse intake of nutrients.

3. Incorporate plant-based proteins like tofu, tempeh, beans, and lentils into meals and snacks.

4. Choose healthy fats like avocado, nuts, seeds, and olive oil for cooking and dressing.

5. Limit consumption of processed foods, refined grains, and added sugars.

6. Enjoy occasional servings of lean meats, poultry, or fish if desired, but prioritize plant-based meals.

7. Be mindful of portion sizes and listen to your body's hunger and fullness cues.

8. Experiment with plant-based cooking techniques and recipes to discover new flavors and textures.

9. Stay hydrated by drinking plenty of water throughout the day.

10. Focus on long-term sustainability and balance rather than strict adherence to rules, allowing for flexibility and enjoyment in your eating habits.

Ornish Diet:

Definition:

The Ornish diet, developed by Dr. Dean Ornish, is a low-fat, plant-based eating plan designed to prevent and reverse heart disease and promote overall health and well-being. It emphasizes whole, unprocessed foods such as fruits, vegetables, whole grains, legumes, and limited amounts of low-fat dairy and plant-based proteins. The diet also encourages regular exercise, stress management, and social support as part of a holistic approach to health.

Ingredients:

- Plant-Based Foods: Fruits, vegetables, whole grains, legumes, nuts, seeds.

- Low-Fat Dairy: Skim milk, low-fat yogurt, cottage cheese (in moderation).

- Lean Proteins: Tofu, tempeh, beans, lentils, chickpeas, edamame.

- Healthy Fats (in moderation): Avocado, nuts, seeds, olive oil.

- Occasional Fish (optional): Fatty fish like salmon, trout, sardines (in moderation).

Instructions/How to Prepare:

1. Base meals around plant-based foods such as fruits, vegetables, whole grains, legumes, nuts, and seeds.

2. Include a variety of colorful fruits and vegetables to ensure a diverse intake of nutrients.

3. Choose low-fat dairy products like skim milk, low-fat yogurt, and cottage cheese in moderation.

4. Incorporate plant-based proteins like tofu, tempeh, beans, and lentils into meals and snacks.

5. Limit consumption of added fats and oils, opting for healthier sources like avocado, nuts, seeds, and olive oil.

6. Minimize intake of animal products, particularly high-fat meats and full-fat dairy.

7. Focus on whole, unprocessed foods and avoid processed and refined foods.

8. Practice stress management techniques such as meditation, yoga, or deep breathing exercises.

9. Engage in regular physical activity, aiming for at least 30 minutes of moderate exercise most days of the week.

10. Cultivate a supportive social network and prioritize meaningful connections with friends and loved ones for overall well-being.

TLC Diet (Therapeutic Lifestyle Changes):

Definition:

The TLC diet is a heart-healthy eating plan designed to reduce cholesterol levels and lower the risk of heart disease. It emphasizes reducing intake of saturated fat and dietary cholesterol while focusing on consuming a variety of nutrient-rich foods, including fruits, vegetables, whole grains, lean proteins, and healthy fats. The diet also encourages regular physical activity and other lifestyle modifications to promote heart health.

Ingredients:

- Fruits: Berries, apples, oranges, bananas, grapes, etc.

- Vegetables: Leafy greens, broccoli, carrots, bell peppers, tomatoes, etc.

- Whole Grains: Oats, barley, quinoa, brown rice, whole wheat bread, whole grain pasta.

- Lean Proteins: Skinless poultry, fish, seafood, tofu, beans, lentils.

- Healthy Fats: Avocado, nuts, seeds, olive oil, fatty fish like salmon.

- Low-Fat or Fat-Free Dairy: Skim milk, low-fat yogurt, reduced-fat cheese.

- Herbs and Spices: Basil, oregano, garlic, turmeric, cinnamon, etc.

Instructions/How to Prepare:

1. Limit intake of saturated fats, trans fats, and dietary cholesterol by choosing lean proteins, low-fat dairy products, and healthy fats.

2. Focus on consuming a variety of colorful fruits and vegetables for essential vitamins, minerals, and antioxidants.

3. Choose whole grains over refined grains for added fiber and nutrients.

4. Incorporate lean proteins such as poultry, fish, tofu, beans, and lentils into meals and snacks.

5. Use healthy fats like avocado, nuts, seeds, and olive oil for cooking and dressing.

6. Limit consumption of processed foods, sugary snacks, and high-fat meats.

7. Be mindful of portion sizes to avoid overeating, especially with calorie-dense foods.

8. Read food labels to identify hidden sources of saturated and trans fats, sodium, and added sugars.

9. Stay hydrated by drinking plenty of water throughout the day.

10.   Engage in regular physical activity, aiming for at least 30 minutes of moderate exercise most days of the week to complement dietary changes and promote overall heart health.

FODMAP Diet (Fermentable Oligosaccharides, Disaccharides, Monosaccharides, and Polyols):

Definition:

The FODMAP diet is a therapeutic approach to managing symptoms of irritable bowel syndrome (IBS) and other gastrointestinal disorders. It involves temporarily reducing or eliminating certain types of carbohydrates that are poorly absorbed in the small intestine and can ferment in the colon, leading to gas, bloating, abdominal pain, and other digestive symptoms. The diet consists of three phases: elimination, reintroduction, and personalization.

Ingredients:

- Low-FODMAP Fruits: Berries, citrus fruits, bananas, grapes, kiwi, etc.

- Low-FODMAP Vegetables: Leafy greens, carrots, bell peppers, zucchini, potatoes, etc.

- Low-FODMAP Grains: Quinoa, rice (white and brown), oats (gluten-free), etc.

- Low-FODMAP Proteins: Chicken, turkey, fish, eggs, tofu, tempeh, firm tofu, etc.

- Low-FODMAP Dairy: Lactose-free milk, lactose-free yogurt, hard cheeses (e.g., cheddar), etc.

- Low-FODMAP Fats and Oils: Olive oil, coconut oil, butter (in moderation), etc.

- Herbs and Spices: Basil, oregano, ginger, turmeric, cinnamon, etc.

Instructions/How to Prepare:

1. Start with the elimination phase, during which high-FODMAP foods are eliminated from the diet for 2-6 weeks to reduce symptoms.

2. Base meals around low-FODMAP foods such as fruits, vegetables, grains, proteins, and fats that are well-tolerated.

3. Gradually reintroduce high-FODMAP foods one at a time in small portions to identify trigger foods and tolerance levels.

4. Keep a food and symptom diary to track reactions to specific foods and help identify patterns.

5. Personalize the diet by incorporating a variety of low-FODMAP foods that are well-tolerated and avoiding or limiting high-FODMAP foods that trigger symptoms.

6. Be mindful of portion sizes and avoid overeating, as consuming large quantities of even low-FODMAP foods can exacerbate symptoms.

7. Consider working with a registered dietitian experienced in the FODMAP diet to ensure proper implementation and guidance throughout the process.

8. Stay hydrated by drinking plenty of water throughout the day to support digestive health.

9. Experiment with cooking methods and recipes to add flavor and variety to meals while adhering to the low-FODMAP guidelines.

10. Monitor symptoms regularly and adjust your diet as needed to manage symptoms effectively and improve overall quality of life.

Pescatarian Diet:

Definition:

The pescatarian diet is a plant-based eating pattern that includes fish and seafood but excludes other animal meats such as poultry, beef, and pork. It's a flexible approach to eating that emphasizes plant foods such as fruits, vegetables, whole grains, legumes, nuts, and seeds, while also incorporating fish and seafood for protein and essential nutrients like omega-3 fatty acids.

Ingredients:

- Fish and Seafood: Salmon, trout, tuna, mackerel, shrimp, scallops, etc.

- Plant-Based Foods: Fruits, vegetables, whole grains, legumes, nuts, seeds.

- Dairy and Eggs: Milk, cheese, yogurt, eggs (optional, depending on individual preferences).

- Healthy Fats: Avocado, olive oil, nuts, seeds.

- Herbs and Spices: Basil, oregano, garlic, turmeric, ginger, etc.

Instructions/How to Prepare:

1. Base meals around plant-based foods such as fruits, vegetables, whole grains, legumes, nuts, and seeds.

2. Incorporate fish and seafood into meals as the primary source of protein.

3. Choose fatty fish like salmon, mackerel, and trout for their omega-3 fatty acids.

4. Include dairy products and eggs if desired and tolerated, as they provide additional protein and nutrients.

5. Use healthy fats like avocado, olive oil, nuts, and seeds for cooking and dressing.

6. Experiment with a variety of cooking methods, such as grilling, baking, steaming, and sautéing, to enhance flavor and texture.

7. Be mindful of portion sizes and aim for balanced meals that include a variety of food groups.

8. Opt for whole, minimally processed foods and limit intake of processed and refined foods.

9. Stay hydrated by drinking plenty of water throughout the day.

10. Consider supplementing with vitamin B12 and vitamin D if fish and seafood are the primary sources of these nutrients in the diet.

Here's a 31-day meal plan from "The Complete Diabetic Cookbook for Beginners":

CHAPTER 12
31 DAYS MEAL PLAN

Week 1:

Day 1:

- Breakfast: Scrambled eggs with spinach and mushrooms.
- Lunch: Grilled chicken salad with mixed greens and tomatoes.
- Dinner: Baked salmon with roasted asparagus.

Day 2:

- Breakfast: Greek yogurt with berries and a sprinkle of nuts.
- Lunch: Turkey and cheese wrap with lettuce and mustard.
- Dinner: Stir-fried tofu with broccoli and brown rice.

Day 3:

- Breakfast: Oatmeal with sliced bananas and a drizzle of honey.
- Lunch: Tuna salad with cucumber slices.
- Dinner: Grilled shrimp skewers with zucchini noodles.

Day 4:

- Breakfast: Whole grain toast with avocado and poached eggs.

- Lunch: Spinach and feta salad with balsamic vinaigrette.

- Dinner: Baked chicken thighs with roasted Brussels sprouts.

Day 5:

- Breakfast: Cottage cheese with sliced peaches.

- Lunch: Turkey and vegetable stir-fry.

- Dinner: Baked cod with lemon and herbs, served with steamed green beans.

Week 2:

Day 6:

- Breakfast: Smoothie with almond milk, spinach, and berries.

- Lunch: Turkey lettuce wraps with hummus.

- Dinner: Beef stir-fry with broccoli and cauliflower rice.

Day 7:

- Breakfast: Whole grain waffles with Greek yogurt and berries.

- Lunch: Chicken Caesar salad.

- Dinner: Grilled salmon with roasted sweet potatoes.

Day 8:

- Breakfast: Scrambled eggs with tomatoes and cheese.

- Lunch: Turkey and cheese sandwich on whole grain bread.

- Dinner: Stir-fried tofu with mixed vegetables and quinoa.

Day 9:

- Breakfast: Yogurt with mixed berries and a sprinkle of nuts.

- Lunch: Spinach and feta stuffed chicken breast.

- Dinner: Baked tilapia with steamed asparagus.

Day 10:

- Breakfast: Chia seed pudding with almond milk and sliced almonds.

- Lunch: Turkey and avocado wrap with lettuce and tomato.

- Dinner: Beef chili with kidney beans and diced tomatoes.

Week 3:

Day 11:

- Breakfast: Smoothie bowl with mango, banana, and granola.

- Lunch: Chicken and vegetable kebabs with Greek salad.

- Dinner: Baked chicken breast with roasted cauliflower.

Day 12:

- Breakfast: Whole grain toast with almond butter and sliced apples.

- Lunch: Tuna salad with mixed greens and cucumber.

- Dinner: Grilled shrimp with quinoa and roasted Brussels sprouts.

Day 13:

- Breakfast: Greek yogurt with sliced strawberries and a drizzle of honey.

- Lunch: Turkey and cheese roll-up with lettuce and mustard.

- Dinner: Stir-fried tofu with bell peppers and snap peas.

Day 14:

- Breakfast: Scrambled eggs with spinach and mushrooms.

- Lunch: Caprese salad with tomatoes, mozzarella, and basil.

- Dinner: Baked salmon with steamed broccoli.

Day 15:

- Breakfast: Cottage cheese with pineapple chunks.

- Lunch: Turkey and vegetable stir-fry.

- Dinner: Beef stir-fry with broccoli and brown rice.

Week 4:

Day 16:

- Breakfast: Smoothie with almond milk, spinach, and berries.
- Lunch: Turkey lettuce wraps with hummus.
- Dinner: Grilled chicken breast with roasted sweet potatoes.

Day 17:

- Breakfast: Whole grain waffles with Greek yogurt and berries.
- Lunch: Chicken Caesar salad.
- Dinner: Baked cod with lemon and herbs, served with quinoa.

Day 18:

- Breakfast: Scrambled eggs with tomatoes and cheese.
- Lunch: Turkey and cheese sandwich on whole grain bread.
- Dinner: Stir-fried tofu with mixed vegetables and cauliflower rice.

Day 19:

- Breakfast: Yogurt with mixed berries and a sprinkle of nuts.
- Lunch: Spinach and feta stuffed chicken breast.
- Dinner: Baked tilapia with steamed asparagus.

Day 20:

- Breakfast: Chia seed pudding with almond milk and sliced almonds.
- Lunch: Turkey and avocado wrap with lettuce and tomato.
- Dinner: Beef chili with kidney beans and diced tomatoes.

Week 5:

Day 21:

- Breakfast: Smoothie bowl with mango, banana, and granola.
- Lunch: Chicken and vegetable kebabs with Greek salad.
- Dinner: Baked chicken breast with roasted cauliflower.

Day 22:

- Breakfast: Whole grain toast with almond butter and sliced apples.
- Lunch: Tuna salad with mixed greens and cucumber.
- Dinner: Grilled shrimp with quinoa and roasted Brussels sprouts.

Day 23:

- Breakfast: Greek yogurt with sliced strawberries and a drizzle of honey.

- Lunch: Turkey and cheese roll-up with lettuce and mustard.

- Dinner: Stir-fried tofu with bell peppers and snap peas.

Day 24:

- Breakfast: Scrambled eggs with spinach and mushrooms.

- Lunch: Caprese salad with tomatoes, mozzarella, and basil.

- Dinner: Baked salmon with steamed broccoli.

Day 25:

- Breakfast: Cottage cheese with pineapple chunks.

- Lunch: Turkey and vegetable stir-fry.

- Dinner: Beef stir-fry with broccoli and brown rice.

Week 6:

Day 26:

- Breakfast: Smoothie with almond milk, spinach, and berries.

- Lunch: Turkey lettuce wraps with hummus.

- Dinner: Grilled chicken breast with roasted sweet potatoes.

Day 27:

- Breakfast: Whole grain waffles with Greek yogurt and berries.

- Lunch: Chicken Caesar salad.

- Dinner: Baked cod with lemon and herbs, served with quinoa.

Day 28:

- Breakfast: Scrambled eggs with tomatoes and cheese.
- Lunch: Turkey and cheese sandwich on whole grain bread.
- Dinner: Stir-fried tofu with mixed vegetables and cauliflower rice.

Day 29:

- Breakfast: Yogurt with mixed berries and a sprinkle of nuts.
- Lunch: Spinach and feta stuffed chicken breast.
- Dinner: Baked tilapia with steamed asparagus.

Day 30:

- Breakfast: Chia seed pudding with almond milk and sliced almonds.
- Lunch: Turkey and avocado wrap with lettuce and tomato.
- Dinner: Beef chili with kidney beans and diced tomatoes.

Day 31:

- Breakfast: Smoothie bowl with mango, banana, and granola.
- Lunch: Chicken and vegetable kebabs with Greek salad.

- Dinner: Baked chicken breast with roasted cauliflower.

THE END